Magic Ear Kids

Stories of Parenting a Child with Hearing Loss

Joey Lynn Resciniti

ISBN-13: 978-1978442528
ISBN-10: 1978442521

DEDICATION

For Julia

ACKNOWLEDGMENTS

I am grateful to my husband and daughter for their patience and support of my writing. To the audiologists, speech therapists, teachers, mentors, and parents that have helped us along over the years… thank you!

A NOTE ON TERMINOLOGY

My daughter, Julia, has hearing loss. Nine years ago, when she was first diagnosed, I sometimes used the term "hearing impaired." I was quickly notified by an adult blogger with hearing loss that no one wants to be "impaired." It has a negative connotation.

So, I deliberately adopted "hard of hearing" and "hearing loss" as the descriptors around our house. Julia would tell you she has a hard time hearing without her hearing aids.

Some families facing the same level of moderate to severe hearing loss use the word "deaf." In the beginning, I didn't put much thought into the semantics of it all.

I began to form an opinion personally on a family trip to Niagara Falls. Our hotel was on the 49th floor. The view was incredible and worthwhile even with a ridiculously long elevator ride to the ground floor swimming pool.

After an evening swim, Julia was dripping wet and

without her hearing aids in the elevator. We know a few signs and Julia can hear loud speech at close range. We get along pretty well at the pool and while waiting to dry off.

A middle-aged man got in the elevator and began to make friendly small talk with Julia. It was obvious that she'd just been swimming. He was trying to ask her if she liked the water slide. She did not respond.

"She's deaf," my husband explained.

I nearly gasped. Immediately, I felt like screaming, "She is not. She is hard of hearing."

The man continued talking. Tim leaned over to repeat the questions so Julia could answer. I stood back, feeling strange about the bizarre knee-jerk reaction I'd just experienced.

"It was just easier to say 'deaf,'" Tim explained later when I revealed my innermost ravings on the topic. I agreed, all the while aware that I would have given the man an educational presentation occupying the entire length of the elevator ride.

Through the years, I've attended many workshops, participated in conferences, volunteered for parent panels, and served on the board of directors for a parent support organization. These experiences drove home the point that we should all be using "people-first" language. This is to say that you literally list the person before the disability. For example, you'd say "person with hearing loss" rather than "hearing impaired person."

In addition to "people-first" language, hearing loss has its own distinctions between people that identify as Deaf and people that have some level of deafness. Deaf with a capital "D" is a culture with its own language (American Sign Language or ASL) and customs. Julia does not identify herself as Deaf.

Many of the essays in this book were written years ago while our understanding of hearing loss was still developing. At times, the term "hearing impaired" may be used and there may be instances where "people-first" language is not used. This reflects the evolution of our family's experience with hearing loss and perhaps the maturity gained from years of experience with hearing, speaking, and living with loss.

IT BEGINS IN THE BOOTH

By the time we made it to the audiologist's booth at Children's Hospital's northern satellite office in 2008, I had already come to terms with my daughter having some level of hearing loss. Or maybe not. The thing was, I didn't understand hearing the way I do today. In the time between scheduling the appointment and having it, there was a considerable amount of family discussion.

"Well, she heard THAT," we'd say of some noise. Then she'd turn her back and I would call, "Julia!" She wouldn't even flinch. That was my major sign.

The night before the appointment, I had a heart-to-heart with my husband. I told him that if she could hear normally then we had big problems. Julia was engaged and interested in a lot of things. Talking wasn't one of them. For a year of speech therapy in our home there had been little gains, but on the night before our diagnosis, I felt like I was banging my head off the wall. She had become completely disinterested in speech.

During the test, Julia sat on my lap. The audiologist closed us into the soundproof booth. We waited in eerie silence as she went into the other room to watch us through a small window as whirling whistles played over speakers. The sounds were very loud in the beginning. When Julia turned toward the speaker that was making the sound, she was rewarded with a little mechanical character that lit up and did a dance.

As the sounds got quieter, I got a heavy feeling in my stomach. *She's failing pretty bad*, I thought.

But even then, I had strange conflicted feelings. She was just a baby (in a month she'd turn three-years-old). Maybe she just didn't like the dancing bear. My brain couldn't choose which disability I preferred for my daughter: hearing loss or that other thing. The other thing being whatever was keeping her from learning to talk. But maybe there was no other thing, and that was where my hopes rested.

About now I would like to go back and shake the past me. I would tell her it will be okay, this is going to work out. But that day, the whole thing seemed like it was falling apart. I thought she was healthy and she wasn't. I thought I had done a good job being pregnant and I obviously hadn't.

The audiologist leaned into the microphone and told me she was coming over to our room.

I took a deep breath and very specifically warned myself not to cry. "I found a moderate hearing loss in both ears," the audiologist said.

There was a lot more information that day. She used

little rectangular block headphones to transmit the sound directly to the nerves. She could tell that this was a nerve problem, not some little tube that was too small in my baby's ear. I was told that it is not uncommon for a newborn to pass a hearing screening, like mine did, and then find something later.

She reassured me that we'd found it sooner rather than later. That intense speech therapy would catch her up. I had gone inconsolable and was trying to hide my tears in a tissue.

The next few months were tough. We scheduled an ABR test and had to cancel it due to an ear infection. In an **A**uditory **B**rainstem **R**esponse (ABR) test, they sedate the child and play a series of clicks while measuring brain activity. This test is often done for young children to confirm their hearing loss before they're fitted for hearing aids. If the child is old enough to give "reliable and repeatable behavioral test results," the audiologist might not need to put the child through the additional testing. Sedation is necessary after babies are about five months old as the child must be in a very deep sleep for the duration of the test, but some younger babies can have the test while they sleep naturally.

Julia needed the sedated ABR and the added delay in having it gave us extra time to debate the results of the booth test. I was pretty confident, since I was there, that the audiologist knew what she was talking about.

Still, there were those sounds Julia could hear. Our family was not ready to accept the diagnosis and kept questioning the booth test.

On the day of the rescheduled ABR, Julia's ears were clear and healthy. I was with her as she was prepped for the procedure. She had an IV and when it was time for the nurse to hold a mask over her tiny face to put her under, it was my job to hold her tight. I cried because she trusted me, trusted me to let strangers gas her. She fell limp in my arms, and I placed her in a hospital crib.

The waiting room was a dismal wakeup call. My husband and I were vaguely aware of families waiting on much dire results than confirmation of the impairment of one sense. Open heart surgery and cancer treatments had parents together, waiting in that room. Our moment in that place was just a little hiccup in the life of a healthy child.

Julia awoke from her anesthesia. We carried her home with the news that the booth test results were accurate. By then the diagnosis was somewhat easier to process and I set to work managing the appointments and paperwork that would eventually help my daughter speak and thrive.

Moderate sensorineural hearing loss became part of our story that day in the booth.

ORIGIN UNKNOWN

Julia was a full-term baby born exactly one week before her due date. She was healthy and perfect. She passed her newborn hearing screening.

The hospital bassinet had a cabinet underneath where the diapers were stored. If I wasn't very careful with the doors, they would slam loudly. Julia would startle and cry.

At least she can hear, I thought.

I thought about her hearing a lot even before she was born. I used to read to my belly and play music for the baby brain developing within.

I thought that my singing calmed her as an infant.

Then just before she turned three we found out she couldn't hear, not normally anyway. I was devastated. I wanted someone to tell me if she ever heard me. Has she ever heard me sing to her? Has she heard me whisper 'I love you'?

The tests were inconclusive as they often are. The ENT, Ear, Nose, and Throat Specialist, assumes the loss is genetic, but the markers haven't been discovered yet. No one knows if the loss is progressive. No one knows if she could hear when she was a baby.

All of it bothered me. I wanted answers back then. Especially the bit about her hearing potentially getting worse, I really wanted to know about that.

As time goes by, those early years begin to fall into their proper place. I used to think it would mean something to me if she could someday tell me that she heard me when she was a little toddler. Time and distance have shown that she doesn't remember much of anything from her pre-lingual years. Her memories start when she was about four. Everything prior to that comes from pictures and videos. Thankfully, we have a lot of those and in them we look like the happiest people on the planet. So, I think it's safe to give up the late diagnosis guilt.

MEDICAL ASSISTANCE MIRACLE

During the first visit to the booth, the audiologist gave me a tissue (for all my ugly crying) and a packet prepared by Children's Hospital. "Don't worry about anything," she said. "Call this woman, her sole purpose is to handle insurance issues. Pennsylvania is the best place to live if your child needs hearing aids. You won't have to pay for anything."

The packet became a lifeline that gave me something to do as I set out to make up for the time lost by Julia's late diagnosis. First, our family had to be denied Social Security benefits due to our income. Then there was a lengthy form to fill out. Children's recommended writing "MA for Disabled Child" across the top of every page. The form could be faxed, mailed, or delivered in person.

I'm not a fan of downtown Pittsburgh, but I had my mom come to watch Julia and I went into the belly of the beast to the PA Department of Health and Human Services. Parking was hard to come by and when I emerged from the underground garage, I realized there was a solid chance I might never find my car again.

The Department of Health and Human Services was a dank, dreary place. I took a deli counter number and waited to be called by a case worker. Eventually, a Kenyan gentleman made an approximation of my number. I went to his desk and presented the completed Medical Assistance application.

I couldn't understand a word the man said at first. He took the form and indicated he would have it filed. My special Children's Hospital packet said that I should ask for a receipt if I filed the form in person.

"Can I get a receipt?" I asked.
"There is no receipt," he said.
"It says here I'm supposed to ask for a receipt," I said.
"We don't make receipts. There are no receipts," he repeated.

It was in this moment I discovered a new power within myself. I'd been a mother for a few years. I knew that I'd always do whatever I could for my little girl, but I never really felt very empowered until that very moment with the Kenyan, not-native-English speaking, case worker. We had to have this insurance to get my daughter's hearing aids. Any delay in the insurance would keep her from being able to hear and speak. I wasn't going home without a receipt!

So, I just sat and stared at the man.

He shuffled uncomfortably. I could see the change in his face when he realized: *crazy lady ain't going nowhere.*

"I'll go see what I can do," he said.

He walked with two canes under great difficulty and he was gone for an inordinately long time. When he returned, he had a small slip. It was just a printed fax confirmation, but it was a receipt.

I thanked him and began the search for my car.

Within a few days of the definitive ABR test to confirm Julia's hearing levels, a bright yellow Access card came in the mail. A week or so later it was replaced with a more socially acceptable UPMC for You card that paid in full for a pair of hearing aids, ear molds, audiologist check-ups, ENT visits, and all of Julia's routine medical care.

"I've never seen anyone get MA approved this fast," the audiologist commented when we visited her again to order the hearing aids.
"I wouldn't leave without a receipt," I told her. "And I think he had to submit the paperwork to Harrisburg right then, so he could give me something that would get me to leave!"

Medical Assistance has been a miracle. No private insurance would pay for hearing aids even though Julia's hearing loss is deemed educationally handicapping. My kid couldn't hear enough to learn to talk, but in most states, that would have been our problem alone. We would have likely taken a loan and had a hearing aid payment for the rest of our lives. Not so in Pennsylvania.

Pennsylvania kids with all kinds of disabilities are on

Medical Assistance, removing a burden from their families that allows them to focus on caring for the child rather than figuring out a payment plan. There is no income restriction for a qualifying disability. The program has been a blessing for our family and a benefit of living here that will be hard for any other place to top.

BRAND NEW MAGIC EARS

We ordered flesh colored hearing aids with clear ear molds that first time. Julia didn't have much language and truthfully, I was afraid she'd pick some loud color that she'd lose interest in. Her favorite color had changed six times in three years.

The audiologist showed us how to insert a size thirteen battery and talked to us about school accommodations and speech therapy as she programmed the little hearing aids for Julia's specific loss.

I'd thought about the moment she'd first hear with her new hearing aids for the past two months. It was going to be the first time she'd hear my voice. Maybe the first time ever. I wanted to say, "I love you." I wanted to say something nice. Something comforting.

The audiologist worked the molds into her ears and clicked the battery doors shut. Julia's eyes opened wide and her hands clenched on the arms of her chair. She could hear, and she was terrified!

"These are your new magic ears," the audiologist said.

I didn't say anything nice or comforting. I laughed. She looked so adorable, like she was on a roller coaster rather than an office chair. I forgot all about making a grand first speech to her.

Julia's head swiveled to the ceiling. I noticed an obnoxiously loud fan for the first time.

"Do you think she can hear that now?" I asked.
"Yes, that's the trouble with hearing aids. They make everything louder."

On the way home, Julia tried to repeat just about everything we said. At home, we took our dog on the same walk we'd taken every afternoon for the past year. As soon as we got out of the house, Julia ran to edge of a steep hill where a road with a lot of traffic passed below. She wanted to see what all the noise was from.

"Those are cars!" I told her. "You hear the cars!" I was choked up for most of that walk to the park. We had to stop and listen as a man dragged his garbage can over his black top driveway. Every noisy thing that I had never taken the time to notice before was new and interesting.

We were warned that it might be difficult to get Julia to wear her new magic ears. The audiologist suggested being very firm and having her wear the devices during all waking hours. I agreed.

Julia tried to take her aids out once in the car. The squealing gave her away as soon as they were out. I stopped on the side of the road because we were still in our neighborhood where there's no traffic. I got out, opened her car door, and calmly put the hearing aids back in.

"You need to wear your magic ears," I told her.

And from then on, she did.

HEARING LOSS EXPLAINED

Hearing loss has always been difficult to explain to the people around my daughter. I rely heavily on my own past perceptions of the hard of hearing to attempt to understand their difficulty. Before I became educated and intimately acquainted with the workings of the ears, I just didn't understand much about hearing.

Before Julia, the only hard of hearing person I knew was my grandfather. His hearing was destroyed during World War II. He had hearing aids that he wouldn't wear. Our communication with him consisted of yelling at increasing volume and repetition.

Seeing hard of hearing older folks made me think that hearing was sort of "on" or "off". Grand pap used to hear, after the war he didn't. Everything needed to be louder. When Julia was a baby, I knew that she could hear because she responded to some sounds. I really didn't know there could be such an impact from moderate hearing loss. I had no idea of all the things she wasn't hearing.

The first thing the audiologist showed us after the ABR

testing's conclusive result was the "speech banana." This was a confusing bit of information at first. I remember feeling weepy when I saw that whispering and birds singing were so far out of her range. I studied the chart (pictured below) and tried to figure out where Julia's speech approximations came from and how we took so long to diagnose the hearing loss.

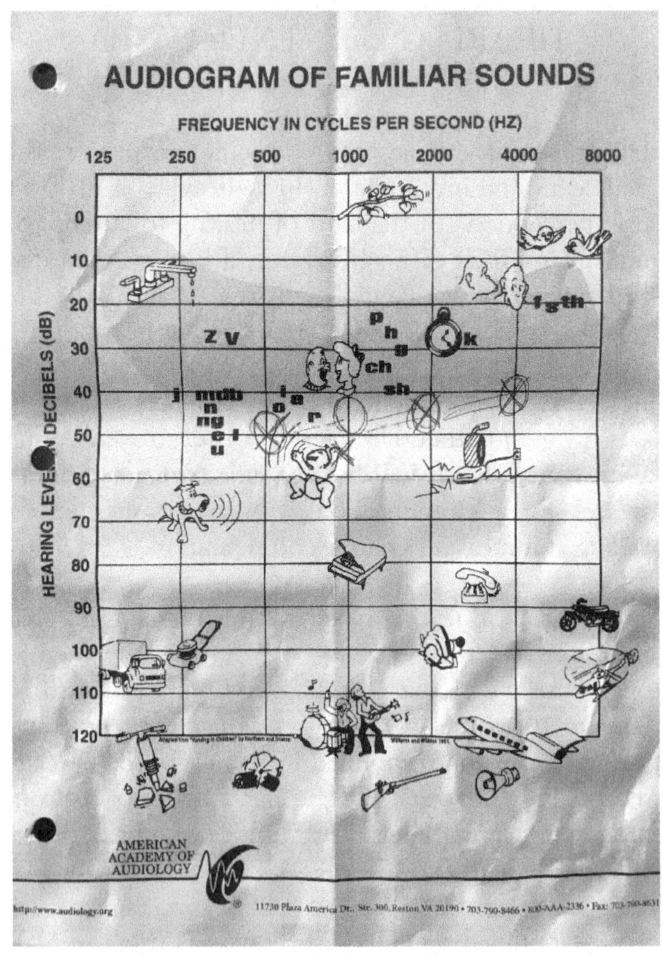

The speech banana was the visual aid for a very quick introduction to hearing loss and the varying levels of severity. Normal hearing is in the 0-20dB range at the top of the banana. Julia's 55 dB loss when she was first diagnosed is marked with X's and O's. All of the speech sounds are above that mark. Theoretically, without hearing aids she can't hear any of those sounds.

Things louder than 55 dB like a dog barking or a piano would be accessible for her without hearing aids. But the tricky part is that it isn't so cut and dry. She wasn't missing all language and hearing dogs barking consistently. There are just too many variables to figure out what her world was like before the hearing aids.

Julia's first set of hearing aids "corrected" her 55dB loss. Aided, Julia was hearing above the banana. Still not as good as normal hearing due to background noise and other interference that I might never understand, but she could hear "normally" and began speaking immediately.

Julia's preschool teachers would ask, "can she hear me?" They saw the hearing aids and assumed she was deaf. I got a lot of experience explaining moderate sensorineural hearing loss in those early days. For a while I didn't even leave home without my speech banana.

THE INEFFECTIVE SPEECH THERAPIST

When Julia was 15-months-old, I became concerned with her speech or the lack of any. She'd babbled a little bit as an infant and then didn't say much until at a year or so she said, "hi."

One time.

No one wanted to admit there was a problem. My husband was even a little defensive about the subject. Grandparents chimed in that she was just a "late talker."

I brought the issue to the pediatrician and she recommended having a multi-disciplinary evaluation by our local early intervention agency, The Alliance for Infants and Toddlers. A case worker for the birth to three program came to the house and determined that Julia qualified for speech therapy. Soon after, a speech language pathologist was coming to the house twice weekly.

L--, the speech therapist, was in her early thirties. She wore trendy square-frame glasses and brought a bag of toys and puzzles with her to each appointment. Something was off about her though and Julia didn't like her.

Julia, a ray of sunshine (I'm not just saying that because I'm her mother), liked everyone. She would smile at the grossest looking people in the grocery store. She was like a baby ambassador to the undeserving humans of the world. When L—showed up, Julia seemed to remember she had something to do in another room. L—couldn't hold her interest and never developed any rapport.

It occurs to me that I might have asked to have a different therapist assigned to our case. I didn't want to offend L—though. She did seem to think she was living out her life's calling. Who am I to point out that she wasn't very good at it?

I've since talked to others that work for the Alliance. They offered assurances that we would have been ignored or reassigned to someone worse. So there's that.

All this time, no one suspected Julia wasn't hearing. Small gains were made in her speech. I learned how to use books to prompt language development rather than simply reading the stories over and over. She developed a vocabulary of 20-30 words and then L—indicated she should start forming two-word sentences and learn more complicated multi-syllable words.

Julia didn't get there.

When I informed L—of the hearing test results, I asked if she could spend her last visits before Julia's third birthday teaching us some sign language to bridge the gap before the hearing aids were dispensed.

"Sure," she said.

L—just didn't do that.

Julia's last session was spent with L—holding her under her arms and hopping her from one floor tile to another while attempting to get her to repeat the syllables in the word "petunia."

"PE – TUNE – YA," she spat as she hopped my darling daughter through our house.

It was one of the most painful things I've seen someone do to my child. If I could go back in time I would boot L—out of my house.

"Let me know how everything turns out," L—said as she left us for the last time.

I didn't do that.

Catching lightning bugs before hearing aids

A Magic Ear Kids blog post from June 27, 2010:

Lightning bugs (fireflies) have been out for several weeks. Our yard is a perfect habitat for them. Julia has been out with the neighborhood girls way past bedtime collecting loads of the things in her buggy box.

She is really interested in the specifics this year. *What do lightning bugs eat? How do they light up?*

I figured I'd put off these important questions long enough one day while we were at my mom's house. I took Julia on my lap to google it once and for all.

Before I opened the browser, I spied an item on the desktop of my mother's computer. It was a video clip called "Lightning Bugs." We watched an eighteen second clip of Julia seeing the blinking insects for the first time. She was about two. She didn't have hearing aids and we didn't know she needed them.

Julia didn't attempt to speak. I listened to myself prompting her. "Look, it's a bug. Can you say BUG? Catch the BUG!" Julia didn't say anything. She raised her small hands and tracked the flashing creature.

We didn't have a video camera back then. I'm almost glad we didn't. The few grainy cell phone/digital camera videos we have are painful for me to watch.

Some are even more painful than this lightning bug one.

There's a video of Julia pretending she's reading stories aloud to me and Tim and his mom. She was approximating speech at that time. Her utterances were combination of a d-sound and vowels.

We thought everything was okay back then. Now that video sounds like a deaf child to me. I wish I'd known then that she needed help. I wish I hadn't spent a whole year frustrating myself and my baby. I wish I could go back to that first night she saw lightning bugs. I'd tell myself to get her hearing tested. I'd tell myself that she's going to be okay and that in three short years she'll say so much more than "bug."

The best I can do now is to forgive myself. I'm doing it one grainy video at a time.

A TOUR OF THE VERY BEST SCHOOL FOR HARD OF HEARING CHILDREN IN THE WHOLE WORLD…AND SORRY, SHE CAN'T GO THERE

At age three, kids graduate from the Alliance for Infants and Toddlers where the lovely L—worked to the Allegheny Intermediate Unit's Project DART. DART (Discovery, Assessment, Referral and Tracking) serves children age three to five.

Not to get bogged down in the intricacies of early intervention in Allegheny County, Pennsylvania, but the transition from the birth-three program to DART is like being shoved out of a 50-story building.

Julia's hearing loss diagnosis came just as she was graduating from the Alliance home-based program and advancing into this adversarial, administrator-eat-parent preschool system. We had to choose an option for her continued speech therapy without knowing what the options were for her continued speech therapy.

At the same time, the DePaul School for Hearing and

Speech was celebrating some important anniversary (it was a multiple of ten to be sure) which led them to sponsor closed captioning for every program on our local ABC affiliate. I was sure to look that school up as soon as hearing loss was identified as an issue. I scheduled a tour and figured all our difficulties would soon melt away.

The DePaul School for Hearing and Speech was all kinds of wonderful. Every room in the building was outfitted with top notch technology, soundproofing, and everything a child with hearing aids could need. Student to teacher ratios were practically like having a private tutor for each kid. Every classroom revealed a new wonder.

"What do we have to do for our daughter to go here?" was asked before we even got to the conference room where I assumed there would be a document to sign over all our worldly possessions in exchange for a semester of preschool.

Instead we were informed that you can't pay to send your child to DePaul. The DART program has to approve and then the Allegheny Intermediate Unit pays for your child to go to DePaul.

That day we had our first lesson on the Individualized Educational Plan (IEP) and least-restrictive environments. We learned that we could fight for placement at DePaul, but it was unlikely to be approved as Julia had moderate hearing loss and didn't demonstrate enough of a delay to require the intensity of DePaul's program.

The staff at DePaul felt convinced that Julia would benefit from their program and should go to their school. They described the other DART options for speech therapy, but nothing could compare to what they offered which was guaranteed success.

I wanted that guarantee more than anything. It became apparent that we needed to entertain the possibility that placement at DePaul might not happen and focus on the other options provided by the DART program. It was a blow to find out our solution wasn't widely accepted as a viable option, but that visit to the very best school in the whole wide world turned out to be an important part of the process. Without it there's no way we'd have known how to get what our daughter needed from the options that were on the menu.

PRIVATE SPEECH THERAPY, THE FIRST IEP MEETING, AND THE BEST TEACHER EVER

The day after Julia's magic ears were first turned on, she started private speech therapy at the Children's Hospital's North campus. It was determined that she would benefit from sessions twice per week. Every sound she learned was drilled and practiced in the tiny office of her speech therapist, E--.

On a few occasions, I would observe through one-way glass with headphones to hear their work. It never failed to make me feel like crying. Whether she was making progress or stalled in a dreaded plateau, the feeling of watching her in that little cube laboring over what should have come without effort made me sad.

The private speech therapy was easy compared to the pending battle for a preschool placement with DART. Armed with information from the DePaul School, I visited the various options which included a preschool program where speech therapy consisted of one therapist with eighteen kids having "circle time" and an odd small speech therapy class where three kids worked with a therapist in a church basement classroom. Neither option was impressive.

The first IEP meeting was attended by an interim teacher of the deaf. She was a personable young girl and it might have been her first IEP meeting as well. She looked at Julia's audiogram and explained that our daughter could hear everything without her hearing aids. I looked at her quizzically for a moment and she exclaimed, "oh, I'm looking at it upside down!"

For three hours we were in a room with the teacher, a speech language pathologist and the director of the DART program, a woman I'll call the S.S. Administrator. S.S. was fierce, and she was not about to place our daughter at DePaul. It was a struggle to get the woman to the meeting in the first place, how we kept her there for that amount of time, I can't recall. We talked through every option and when it was over, we had a speech therapist visiting Julia one day a week at a private preschool and the odd small group speech therapy in the church basement. The meeting ended with our acceptance of subpar services and disappointment.

I'll just have to make up the difference, I thought as I left the meeting, aptly located in a musty church basement.

Soon after, Julia and I started working through the John Tracy Clinic correspondence program. I learned the cues for speech sounds and prompted her to use the ones the speech therapists were working on. We had speech therapy every waking hour of that little girl's life.

The interim teacher of the deaf worked with Julia for just a short while. Her permanent replacement was called Miss A- and she might well have been the one that saved the whole thing.

A graduate of the John Tracy Clinic's graduate program, Miss A-- had been working in the toddler room at the DePaul School on the day we visited. She played with Julia while Tim and I toured the school. Her new position at DART included latitude to create a deaf/hard of hearing playgroup that replaced the strange three on one church basement speech therapy.

Julia went to Miss A--'s magic ear group once a week. She met other kids with hearing loss and developed friendships that continued long past preschool.

Binders full of pictures and stories came home from the class. Adventures with ice skating in shaving cream, monkeys that just wouldn't stop jumping on the bed, and taste tests of green eggs and ham.

We've had occasion to meet many professionals over the years, Miss A-- is the best of the best.

One day, E--, the private therapist came out after their visit and said, "Julia is doing fabulously well. In structured activities, her articulation is perfect."

And then, just eighteen months after the first appointment, our weekly journey to speech therapy ended.

I was a little misty-eyed saying goodbye to our terrific speech therapist that helped us so much in our most difficult parenting hurdle. It was hard to separate the trauma of a change in a long-time routine from the joy of knowing we accomplished just what we wanted to. We achieved our goal – we caught up to normal before kindergarten with time to spare.

Shortly after it was time to say goodbye to Miss A--'s playgroup too. With our mission accomplished, she'd set a standard for teachers of the deaf that might never be equaled.

NO, THEY'RE NOT COCHLEAR IMPLANTS, MAYBE WRITE IT DOWN THIS TIME

The doctors' office I chose before Julia was born had three pediatricians in the practice. I made sure to visit all three during those early weeks when well-baby visits were frequent. I settled on one that I liked better than the others and scheduled appointments with him whenever possible.

Then he retired. So, I would schedule with my second favorite, an older woman with a rough bedside manner. She was the one that referred us to the Alliance for Infants when I expressed concern about Julia's speech at age two.

We returned to her office frequently after Julia got her hearing aids for illnesses and vaccinations.

"Are those cochlear implants?" she asked when she first saw the hearing aids.
"No," I said. "These are hearing aids. Julia has moderate hearing loss, so she just needs hearing aids. Cochlear implants are for more severe losses."

"Oh," the doctor said.

The visit continued, and I felt a little concerned that a medical professional didn't know what a cochlear implant looked like, but everyone has to learn about it sometime. I was glad to help educate her.

On our next visit: "Those are cochlear implants, right?"
And the next: "She has the cochlear implants, doesn't she?"

Every time we went to the pediatrician, the same question about cochlear implants. I offered various explanations and descriptions, hopeful it would jog some memory of our past visits.

It never did.

Finally, I grew tired of feeling like it was our first visit every time. I found a new pediatrician where, amazingly, they recognized Julia's hearing aids right away.

The pediatrician's office is one of the first places Julia recognized a need to advocate for herself. At every visit the nurse wants to use an ear thermometer to take her temperature. Julia doesn't like to have her hearing aids out for even a moment. At first, I'd ask if they could use the old style, under the tongue, thermometer. They're always glad to switch.

Eventually, Julia started asking on her own, "Can you use the under the tongue one instead? I have hearing aids."

It's just a small thing, but it requires confidence. And I'm glad it's happening in an office where the doctors can tell the difference between a hearing aid and a cochlear implant.

TROUBLE WITH A HARD OF HEARING SWIMMER

A Magic Ear Kids blog post from July 6, 2009:

Julia loves to swim. Over four summers she's progressed to have some skill at it. With a pair of goggles, she can swim about six feet under water. She's come a long way from the first trip to the pool when we dipped her tiny baby toes in the water.

Before her hearing loss was discovered at age three, the pool was the same as any other place. It was never any use yelling for her. She was on her way to do what she was going to do. I ran after her and re-directed her. It took all that time for me to realize something, her hearing, was wrong.

Now we live every day with the miracle of her hearing aids. I'm grateful when she stops running because she heard me calling to her. We can tell each other stories. She talks constantly.

When we go to the pool and take out her hearing aids, so she can go in the water, the hearing problem seems progressive. She responds really well at first. It even gives me a thought that she could get by without being aided. As time goes by, she seems to miss more. Lately we've been having tremendous difficulty with her misunderstanding me.

Today was a perfect example. We went for a short swim during which it seemed she could hear everything she needed to. I'm sure there would be no hope of her carrying on a conversation with a stranger, but mom's voice is the most important anyway. We got out of the pool after no more than twenty minutes. The apartment complex doesn't heat the water enough for our liking and Julia needed to warm up.

As we wrapped ourselves in towels, Julia became frustrated that I wasn't putting hers on the way she wanted it. I tried to explain what I was doing. She started to whimper. I conveyed that it was time to go home anyway.

She's been a real stinker about wanting to let her hair air dry. This has always been a point of contention with us. I spent all of last summer trying to minimize the time she spent without her hearing aids so that she could be exposed to as much language as possible. Now that she is doing so well and talking every minute of the day, I figure it will be okay if she spends longer days at the pool and even if she lets her hair air dry.

Once we were home, it took about six tries to get her to understand that she should put on underwear. All of this even though we were standing two feet from each other. She was facing me, and I really think that she'd have gotten this just after her hearing aids came out. I finally had to open her drawer and point.

The hair was still air drying and Julia was having blueberries for a snack. She brought one to me that was all brown and instructed me to eat it. I didn't want to eat it and I told her neither of us should eat it. I threw it into the bushes and she immediately started sobbing. She wanted to eat blueberries. I told her she could still eat the good blueberries. She started into a tantrum.

I decided that enough was enough and I was going for the hair dryer. That did not go over well.

Once the hearing aids were back in, the misunderstanding and the tantrum were soon resolved. Julia remained mad at me for a while because she didn't want her hair dried.

I'm stymied with this issue. I've spoken to her hearing teacher and I've never had a bit of advice other than to make sure she's looking at me when I speak to her. She is looking at me and she's still not getting it.

I think as Julia grows up, she'll be able to compensate for the hearing loss when she's swimming. I hope so, because she has the makings of a tremendous swimmer. Perhaps in the meantime I'll have to learn sign.

ARTICULATING FOR THE PRINCESS

In September of 2009, we really couldn't wait any longer to visit Disney World with our little girl. She'd become hooked on princess movies around her third birthday. As she learned more and more language she used to tell us adorable stories about Beauty and the Beast. "Gaston shoot the bear," she would say. "Gaston make the bear into a rug."

It was a great triumph for her to say that many words in a row.

We planned a five-night vacation and stayed in the value hotel, the All-Star Music Resort. Julia packed several princess dresses and basically owned the place with her light brown curls and general adorableness.

Though speech therapy had progressed well, we were told that certain sounds just didn't "come in" until kids were much older. This was true of the "J" sound and it was predicted that Julia wouldn't be able to say her own name until she was six or seven-years-old.

It seemed like much too long for her to go around

calling herself "Ee-ya" and I didn't so much accept that pronouncement. I kept trying to prompt Julia with the hand cues I'd observed during her speech therapy sessions.

Julia was fairly oblivious to this flaw in her speech until we started meeting princesses.

"What's your name, princess?" Cinderella asked.

Everyone from the characters to the janitors called Julia "princess" in the Magic Kingdom.

"Ee-ya," she would say.

Cinderella looked at me, very confused.

"Julia," I'd say.

This happened with Belle and many others. We were waiting in line to visit six princesses in some sort of royal hall extravaganza. We talked about which ones we would meet, and I told her, "The princesses can't understand your name unless you make your good "J" sound."

She looked at me with her big eyes and placed a finger to her bottom lip. "J--- J--- Julia!" she said.
"That's it!"

Tim was recording just about everything that happened on our trip and so the very first time she said her own name is preserved. She went around to every princess in that room, placed her index finger on her bottom lip, wound up, and announced, "my name is J--, J--, Julia!"

It wasn't long before she was able to produce the sound without the cue and eventually she could do it without getting a run up to it with those first few J's.

She was four-years-old.

THE GIRL WITH THE THINGS IN HER EARS

A Magic Ear Kids blog post from October 13, 2009:

We've never had anyone notice Julia's hearing aids. She usually wears her hair down or "straight" as she calls it. The over-the-ear part is flesh colored and she has clear ear molds. From a distance you can't even see them.

Ballerina hair styles, usually a bun, and close proximity of dancers has led to some commentary on her magic ears during ballet class. After class her teacher told me that one of the other little girls addressed my daughter, "hey girl with the things in her ears." The kids are so *innocent* was the teacher's take on it.

In the car Julia told me that a girl asked last week, "what are those things in your ears?" Julia told her they were "magic ears" and the girl didn't understand so she told her that they help her hear better. My pride in her ability to explain her disability is tempered with an annoyed worry for the future.

Perhaps my experiences of having a pair of really ugly eyeglasses in the first grade are making me think we'll have tough times over this in the future. A boy in my class, Matt, who incidentally did remain our school's resident hottie even into High School, said that my glasses were upside down. They had that kooky stem most commonly seen on old lady glasses. When he got over harping on them being upside down, he latched onto them probably being my grandmother's glasses. Needless to say, I was more comfortable wearing my conformist wire frame glasses from then on.

By Middle School, I was wearing a Milwaukee brace to treat my scoliosis. Kids weren't as mean as adults I encountered during that time.

Julia has no choice. She'll have to wear her hair up sometimes and innocence will soon be a word no longer associated with the kids in her class. I can only hope that her current sunny, resilient personality will carry her through those times when someone tries to make her feel self-conscious.

And that kid in her ballet class better learn her name is Julia.

THE CONSTANT TALKING PHASE

A Magic Ear Kids blog post from October 20, 2009:

When Julia was diagnosed with hearing loss, those close to me tried to pull me out of my devastation by saying, "someday, you'll beg her to be quiet." I would smile, nod, try to suppress the lump in my throat and pray that they were right. They were. I only wish they'd have offered some tactful advice on initiating some quiet time.

In a few days, Julia will have had her hearing aids for 18 months. A short while ago, I was calculating her "length of utterance" to see if she was using three-word sentences. Now we have trouble having on an adult conversation during her waking hours.

She has something to say about everything. She has no internal monologue. She has been in bed for forty-five minutes and she still hasn't stopped talking.

During the day we chat about everything. I do nothing but pay attention to her for the majority of our time together. There's no need to have her stop talking. I've given up luxuries such as having a moment to think my own thoughts.

My husband gets home, and I get the distinct impression he might like to say something. This is because he often tries to speak. Julia barrels right on, she *needs* fifteen different questions pertaining to the plot of Disney's *Hunchback of Notre Dame* answered. "Daddy is trying to tell me something, you have to wait," I tell her. Her sad little face looks like someone just shot our dog.

It seems hopeless in the daily grind that she'll someday be able to modulate her talking. Then I remind myself of the tiny signs of growth in this area: that she doesn't interrupt when I'm reading stories to her, that she can wait while Daddy tells his story. Someday I'll be begging her to tell me what she's thinking. Moments of silence are coming soon!

One thing I've gained from parenting a hearing impaired kid is a supreme appreciation of her speech. We waited such a long time for her to sing us a song or tell us a story, every word she says (and there are so many) is that much more special.

THE FM FIGHT

A Magic Ear Kids blog post from November 12, 2009:

In the time since Julia's hearing loss was diagnosed I've learned much about assistive technology. Here in PA, the county provides her with an FM System that transmits the teacher's voice directly to her hearing aids. The teacher wears a necklace-type transmitter that they simply power ON to use. It's handy in noisy classrooms or when they sing songs with background music. It really helps her. Unfortunately, a great deal of my newfound knowledge pertains to the resistance/inability of preschool staff to use the technology.

In our last preschool, I could find no other excuse than the age of the staff. There were three of the most kind, attentive, wonderful women in her classroom every day. They seemed to go the extra mile for the kids. They just couldn't figure out Julia's FM system. The thing has one button. I showed them how to use it. A hearing support teacher showed them. They didn't think she needed it. Finally, I threatened that if they couldn't figure it out, I would take her to a new school.

Now we're at a new school in a new county. The teacher, a former second grade teacher, was quite familiar with FM. She's used it before. Everything should be copacetic, or so I thought.

Last week, I picked up my lovely daughter and she says, "Mommy, what was that sound?" I hadn't heard anything.
"I didn't hear anything, sweetie. How was your day?" I asked.
"It's my FM," she says, very matter of fact. I look in her backpack that she had just pitched onto the front seat of the car. There inside is her FM packed inside a freezer bag, still powered on. Way to go new preschool!

Now that she's older, these inattentive dolts give her an opportunity to practice her self-advocacy skills. I told her to remind the teachers to turn off the transmitter at the end of the day. She gave me a whole breakdown, "Mommy, when it has numbers it's on. When it has no numbers, it's off."

Just listen to the four-year-old, everything will be okay.

CONSTANT CONCERN IN AN EAR-CENTRIC HOUSEHOLD

A Magic Ear Kids blog post from December 6, 2009:

During preschool on Thursday, I got a phone call. Julia's hearing aids were beeping. There was palpable anxiety in the voice of the go-between chosen to call mom for the teacher. I told her there are batteries in the classroom. I told her where the batteries are located in the classroom. I tried to calm her a little by explaining how to open the battery door. I gave them the option to call me back if they couldn't perform the operation and I would drive back to school and do it.

They never called back. They were able to figure it out. Julia gets in the car after school with the story already barreling out at me. They changed my magic ear battery! Just the left one! I checked and graded them a "B" on putting the aid back in for her. No one gets all of the nooks and crannies lined up like mama does.

This is the first time we've had one go down when I wasn't around. She survived.

But a related issue has popped up since our last

audiologist appointment. The result of that visit on the Monday before Thanksgiving was that Julia is having fluctuations of 5 to 10 dB at a few frequencies. Next time we have to make her wear the ear plugs she despises to try and get consistent readings. For the last three appointments, at Julia's request, she's been wearing headphones. The audiologist thinks this is messing us up. Thankfully, she believes the hearing is stable, but perhaps the headphones are shifting and impacting the results.

The audiologist took the hearing aids for a long time to check the programming. She returned them to us with "fresh" programming and explained that tweaking the programming each time can cause "compression ratios" and stuff to get messed up. She noted that we might hear a difference during our listening check.

I thought that I couldn't possibly notice a difference. I just confirm that they're on and don't sound crackly. But they sound wonderful. Clear and maybe louder and just plain better than before.

Since the "fresh" program we've had two sets of batteries die after only three days. Usually batteries last for at least two weeks. Occasionally we come across some wonder batteries that will last a month. Three days is not a good lifespan.

The FM will draw more power, but if that is the case we should have been seeing a problem since the start of school. We're left to wonder about the super-clear sound being some kind of hyper-power drainer. And my battery tester doesn't really work so what if Julia is false reporting low battery beeps?

All I think about is ears.

Then at bedtime Thursday night, her right ear was hurting. Ear pain about a week after a mild cold. Ugh! The next days found me with my head cocked, listening intently for the tell-tale slushy speech. Thankfully, the pain was a fluke or went away, but I'm still worrying over those ears.

All I ever think about is ears!

LEARNING TO READ IS NOTHING LIKE EASY

A hearing professional once described the mind of a child with hearing loss to me as a "swiss cheese brain." This is to say that there are holes in the child's understanding, but no one can predict what information those holes should have contained. Kids show weakness years into their elementary education with rhyming and alphabetization. It seems those things that a typically hearing child would pick up through incidental learning have to be explicitly taught to a kid with hearing loss.

So, it was that I undertook to teach Julia to read before the start of kindergarten. Literacy is a huge issue in the hearing loss community. Reading is so intertwined with sound and speech. I wasn't confident that the kindergarten program would be entirely successful, and I was committed to putting my daughter at an advantage rather than waiting for her to qualify for extra help when she found herself at a disadvantage.

The reading program I purchased used the word "easy" right in the title. Since we'd already conquered identification of upper and lower-case letters and Julia was well versed in many phonetic sounds from her years of speech therapy, some of the early lessons were not difficult. It was when we slugged through the increasingly challenging words, sentences, and passages that she decided it was a bit more work than she was interested in doing. The lessons were advertised as 15-minute, easily digestible, non-threatening chunks. They turned into 45-minute disagreements complete with ultimatums and tears.

I insisted on those lessons every day that winter even with the gnashing of teeth they were sure to bring. Julia started kindergarten with a firm foundation. She was reading fluently, faster than most of her peers. By third grade, testing showed she was reading at an eighth-grade level.

Looking back, it would have been great to teach her to read without any tears, but I don't regret my determination.

Reading to Supplement Hearing

A Magic Ear Kids blog post from January 17, 2010:

Julia is on a break from preschool. She went to the first school for a whole year. We moved, and she went to a second preschool for a half year. We moved again, and a third preschool was not something I was interested in doing. She gets a two-hour hearing impaired play group once a week and has her dance classes.

Other than that, it's the school of mommy.

Tim thought it would be great for an added method of communication if she could read. Julia thinks it would be great if she could read. I know how to read.

I purchased a reading program on Amazon. *Teach Your Child to Read in 100 Easy Lessons* requires a bit of reading on the part of the parent before beginning. The lessons are short and by building each day on the skills of the previous lesson, they are pretty easy.

Years of speech therapy are paying dividends in the little tasks of our reading lessons. Julia has been associating letters with sounds during intense speech therapy. She already knows a lot of sounds. She has the ability to listen to herself sounding out a word and easily connect it to the printed word. We're thrilled to have this strength that the past years of hard work have given our daughter.

The lessons have also shown a great weakness in rhyming. She simply isn't getting it. Perhaps the speech therapy has caused her to connect words by their beginning sounds. It's been a rough couple of weeks getting her to listen to the ending sounds.

I have no way of knowing whether our troubles are in any way related to hearing loss. I am glad that we've started building reading skills early. I look forward to supplementing her hearing with printed words. Someday she'll be able to watch her favorite movies with closed captions if she chooses. She'll read the lyrics of a song and see the names of roads on the GPS. She'll know that even though it sounds like "Ghost Mustard", it truly is "Ghost Busters" they're singing.

Reading will give her an extra tool to use in decoding the world.

Literacy skills in children with hearing loss

A Magic Ear Kids blog post from February 7, 2010:

Julia and I are one month into our 100 easy lessons that will ultimately teach her to read. As we worked through the tasks in the very well-planned lessons, I found a weakness in Julia's understanding of rhyming and wondered if this was in any way attributed to her hearing loss. She is really insistent on matching the beginnings of words rather than the end.

Over the past weeks we've made progress. She now remembers some rhyming words, but I don't think she's really getting it yet. A listing of skills that develop during kindergarten indicates rhyming is an emergent skill for the five to six-year-old set.

Even if that is the case, some skills take more time for my daughter to master. She has some difficulty with what I would term her auditory memory. Learning a new word or the name of a playmate she's just met takes a lot of practice and repetition. If she mishears a word and pronounces it improperly there can be a whole extra level added to the process. Last summer, Julia was insistent her new friend was Kayton. The name was Peyton. We ended up writing it on a note card, so we could point to it when we tried to say the name. Peyton with a popper sound.

It was because of this concern and the debate over its

cause that I picked up an old copy of *The Volta Review* published in the fall of 2008. I'd been saving it to read sometime and given its title: "Emergent Literacy Skills During Early Childhood in Children With Hearing Loss: Strengths and Weaknesses;" there's no time like the present.

The study involved 44 children age four to six, all with more hearing loss than my daughter. Some of the children used cochlear implants and some had hearing aids. All had access to sound and had "some speech perception skills."

Various tests were used over the course of one school year to measure different literacy skills. In the rhyming test, the children had to pick the picture of the word that rhymed with the target word. The findings revealed that the hard of hearing kids "progressed on some phonological awareness skills (alliteration, blending, and elision) but not on others (rhyming, syllable segmentation)." This was over the course of the yearlong study.

The good news is that hard of hearing kids were on par with typically hearing children when it came to recognizing the letters of the alphabet and common written words.

The bad news is that vocabulary developed more slowly. This was attributed to typical children acquiring vocabulary incidentally. Hard of hearing children must have more direct instruction to remember new words.

The hard of hearing children "performed poorly,

particularly on recognition of rhyming words." It goes on to say this task was the toughest for their study participants.

Their speculative conclusion as to why this might be so is that "in speech therapy, children are taught that 'sounding the same' refers to minimal pairs that share the same phonemes. This might result in confusion if children are told by adults that two words rhyme because they 'sound the same at the end.'" They continued to hypothesize that often teachers (and parents) assume that a child is learning rhyming because nursery rhymes and Dr. Seuss are regularly being read.

The recommendation: more repetition and slower instruction.

This study supported my conclusion that rhyming is tougher for a hard of hearing child. We've been grouping words for years because they start with the bitey sound or the popcorn sound. Now I'm asking her to make this leap to listen to the end of the word. She can see that C-A-T and H-A-T rhyme on paper, but she doesn't yet hear it. Her ears need a bit more training.

The literacy skills presented in this study have renewed my campaign to build Julia's vocabulary. Now that she's saying words correctly, we can learn off-the-wall things like "silo" and "turret". Also, our reading lessons are going really well! In just seventy more days, she'll be reading!

Preceding quotes are from:
"Emergent Literacy Skills During Early Childhood in Children With Hearing Loss: Strengths and Weaknesses"
Susan R. Easterbrooks; Ed.D.;
Amy R. Lederberg, Ph.D.;
Elizabeth M. Miller, M.Ed.:
Jessica P. Bergeron, M.Ed.;
and Carol McDonald Connor, Ph.D.

The Art of Reading Aloud

A Magic Ear Kids blog post from April 4, 2010:

This week I attended a program at the DePaul Institute called "The Art of Reading Aloud, Reading Skill Development through Literature." As always, the people at DePaul put on a great event open to all parents/grandparents of kids with hearing loss, not just DePaul families.

A hearty amount of the discussion dealt with building reading comprehension skills. As parents, we should be asking questions to make sure our little ones are understanding what is read. I've been surprised since working through 90 of Julia's reading lessons (*Teach Your Child to Read in 100 Easy Lessons*) how well she can answer questions based on her own reading of simple stories.

When I read to her, it's a challenge for me to think of questions to ask that will help her get to a higher level of thinking about more complex stories. This workshop has made me aware of the times I read without really knowing if she's paying attention.

Now I've been armed with a list of questions to help her uncover deeper meaning and help her draw on her own experiences to understand the story. I'm interested to ask her how she'd have ended some of her favorite stories if she was the author. We're sure to uncover some big ideas and hopefully she's well on the way to becoming a strong reader. I'm really anxious about conquering spelling, but that's a battle for another day!

DEVELOPING A FIRE SAFETY PLAN

A Magic Ear Kids blog post from January 21, 2010:

Julia has a multi-disciplinary evaluation every year as part of the services she receives from the county for her hearing loss. There are all kinds of questions for her and me during a two-hour visit from her certified teacher of the deaf. This time it revealed little in the way of deficiencies which is wonderful.

The teacher did surprise me by asking Julia what she should do in a fire. I think about what we'd do in a fire all the time. I am a constant worrier. I've been thinking through how I would scoop up my baby and flee the house for the past four years.

I've talked about school fire drills with Julia. I've told her that the smoke alarm means that we should leave the house. We leave the house unless it goes off when mommy is cooking, and I tell her it's a false alarm. She surely thinks that the annoying beeps happen only, so I'll go and swat at the ceiling with a dish towel.

But we had to answer this question and we weren't prepared. My daughter, always innovative in her responses, replied that she would put out the fire. Then I corrected her by saying that she should find mommy. I took a moment and realized that we have no escape plan and we would all die of smoke inhalation.

We've moved into our first house where we can be in separate rooms that are too far apart for us to be heard talking to one another. We're going to need to have a fire drill. I'm going to have to train her to leave the house and meet me at the mailbox. I can't rely on my own ability to find her and get her to safety.

It scares me that this snuck up on me so quickly. Here she is almost five. She could be that kid that goes and hides in a closet where we couldn't get to her in time. My worrying brain is in overdrive.

I have some work to do. We need to have one of those family meetings. We need to plan on getting ourselves out of the house and not stopping for Barbie dolls or even the poor dog. Hopefully, next time she's asked my Julia will know that she's not supposed to play hero fire girl.

JOURNEY TO THE CENTER OF THE PARENT SUPPORT GROUP

I was devastated when Julia's hearing loss was discovered. The ordeal had gone on longer for me that anyone else. I prayed every night from her first birthday on for my baby to say one word. "Just one word, God," I prayed. "To let me know she's alright."

Then for years I was mad. Couldn't God have moved me toward getting her hearing tested when she was younger? Would that have been so hard? Existential crisis aside, I sought to sooth my guilt and worry by amassing as much information about the problem as possible. I read every bit of literature I could find on the subject of sensorineural hearing loss, went to a state sponsored parent education workshop, and attended a parent support group meeting. Each activity provided me with endless opportunities for expanding my knowledge and my list of concerns.

Pamphlets and books were written for kids diagnosed as infants. They served to reinforce the importance of making the baby wear hearing aids all day long. They stressed that the first three years are the most important for language development.

The workshop and support group seemed skewed to the parents of kids with profound losses. My child only had a moderate loss. I felt a little sympathy and an overwhelming vibe that I should be skipping around celebrating that she isn't more deaf. "It's just a moderate loss, she'll be fine."

"My kid is as deaf as this table," one Mom announced. She rapped her knuckles on the table for emphasis.

Support group meetings had an element of competition. Often it was in the sheer number of deaf children contained in one family.

"I've got three. Each one is deafer than the next!"

There I was with a toddler, nearly three years old, just diagnosed. I couldn't imagine how she'd ever speak normally. I needed something more than a brush off, "she'll be fine."

She is fine. Even back then, I knew she would be. But if I was approached by someone starting on their own journey as a parent of a child with hearing loss, I hope I would have something more to offer.

It stinks to find out that your child is going to have a life altering, lifelong disability. It's not like wearing eye glasses. Eye glasses for your ears works to describe hearing aids to a preschool classmate, but it's not an adequate analogy for finding out your baby has never properly heard your voice.

Going to all of the IEP meetings, speech therapy, audiologist appointments, ENT appointments, testing, it can be tough. Even though a whole waiting room of parents were waiting on kids in much more serious situations than mine, I still had a tough time when Julia was under anesthesia to have the ABR test that confirmed her hearing loss.

There have been and will always be some problems. I was deeply concerned that there could be teasing about the hearing aids themselves and the speech delay. I'd witnessed a kid in a grocery cart mocking my daughter and asking his dad why she talked like a baby. Once I had to restrain myself from pinning a boy's arm behind his back and whispering, "I'll break your little arm if you ever touch her hearing aids again, got it?"

I've read about adults with the same level of hearing loss as Julia feeling left out at parties and even family dinners. Leaving the table with hurt feelings because they missed the punchline of a joke. It's something we'll have to be cognizant of in the future. It will never go away.

These things aren't covered by a well-meaning catch all, "it will turn out fine." Sometimes better support comes from sharing the things that are tough and how over time it gets easier.

MORE HEARING LOST

A Magic Ear Kids blog post from February 28, 2010:

After a six-week stint of very little activity, Julia and I had a big Thursday. She had magic ear school and an audiologist appointment. Then in the evening I had to go to a transitional meeting to switch her hearing support services from preschool to kindergarten. It was an epic day in the context of our typical home-bound winter schedule.

It goes without saying that I had contracted a cold earlier in the week. I do, in fact, get sick each time I leave my house. I was buzzing on Mucinex with ironic drowsiness mixed in.

Mentally prepared for a quick audiologist appointment where we filled out a form and talked a little, I was already surprised that we were having a hearing test in the booth. The appointment was to order an FM system for our home since the county will take theirs back this summer. I hadn't prepared Julia to do work. I got the stink eye.

An attempt was made at getting Julia to wear the ear insert do-hickeys that she hates. She got her favored headphones back in pretty short order. After each word the audiologist wanted her to identify she turned to me and said, "these are hurting me!" I can't imagine how they hurt her, but the audiologist went back to the headphones. Even imaginary plight can be distracting from sound identification tasks.

Her picture identification is usually strong and steady. I've watched her do this test numerous times and she's a pro. The audiologist says a word, Julia points to the picture, they move on. This day, it was WHAT? HUH? WHAT IS SHE SAYING?

Then it was time for the test where Julia is required to feed a toy animal when she hears a sound. It was exciting this time because a new bunny needed fed realistic looking carrots. Previous tests have used cardboard cutout foods. Julia kept turning around and asking me if I heard the sound. "I didn't hear the sound. Did you hear the sound?"

I didn't hear the sound. It is not played for the benefit of the audience. There was no way to communicate this to my child when she wasn't wearing hearing aids and had big headphones over her ears. I did some strange pantomime and willed her to finish the test.

We went in to get an FM and came out feeling pretty certain Julia has lost 10-15 dB of hearing across the three middle frequencies. This means we're looking at a 70-dB loss in the middle frequencies. Prior to this appointment we were 50-55 dB at all frequencies. Her hearing aids were reprogrammed.

By the next day, Julia had the cold. Her hearing was still very poor even with the added amplification. And even though she'd had a tympanogram and her ears were clear the previous day, I still can't let go of those 10 dB. I'm still hoping they'll come back in the spring. I'm still hoping it's ear wax. I can't let go of the denial even though this isn't the first test that has revealed this extra loss.

By the next week our lives returned to normal. Her hearing seems okay. I'm now waiting on the report to see if it will say "fluctuating" or "progressive" or maybe just "severe."

None are words I wanted to see.

JUST BECAUSE IT PROGRESSED DOESN'T MAKE IT PROGRESSIVE

An additional 10 dB loss in the middle frequencies eventually became a 10-15 dB loss across all frequencies putting Julia into the "severe" range of hearing loss. This was discovered close to her fifth birthday after about two years of hearing aid use.

Never one to just take life as it comes, I developed multiple theories on the change in Julia's hearing and gave myself several years of worry. My worst-case, personal bogeyman, particularly scary theory was that her hearing loss was progressive.

Some genetic disorders lead to progressively decreased hearing sensitivity that sometimes results in complete deafness. Julia was tested for the known genetic markers of disorders that cause hearing loss, progressive and otherwise. She doesn't have any of those genetic markers. We were told her hearing loss is probably genetic, but caused by undiscovered markers. So, the genetic testing really never provided a concrete release from my professional grade anxiety. The experts couldn't tell us one way or another if the hearing loss would ever progress. Losing those 10-15 dB scared me, and I really wanted to find another explanation that didn't involve increasing levels of hearing loss.

My thought experiment continued because if it wasn't progressive hearing loss, it had to be something else. I figured maybe Julia had matured over time and was finally able to accurately demonstrate her level of hearing loss during the booth test. This would mean that the 50-55 dB tests were incorrect. But the ABR agreed with the booth testing and they couldn't both be wrong.

Neither home-grown theory seemed to fit, so I resolved to accept that Julia's hearing loss progressed once and then remained stable. This provided an uneasy comfort right up to the middle of the middle school years. It was then that an email exchange with Julia's audiologist about those long-lost decibels finally gave me some closure. "Sometimes with a change in a child's ear canal size, it may seem as if there is a 10-15 dB change in hearing across the frequency range," the audiologist wrote. "As the ear grows, a little more sound pressure may be needed to detect sound. This will result in what looks like a change in hearing but may just be growth of the ear canal."

Finally, we had an explanation that made sense! That, and seven years of stable audiograms, made me feel better. I was finally able to let go of those decibels and my fear of losing more.

NATIONAL SUPPORT GROUPS AND COMMUNICATION CONTRAVERSY

I signed up for every group I could find as part of my comprehensive program to educate myself about all childhood hearing issues. It wasn't long before I unearthed controversy beyond my wildest imagining. Having no solid allegiances, I sought support from two organizations.

The Alexander Graham Bell Association for the Deaf and Hard of Hearing (AG Bell)

The DePaul School, my first stop after the audiologist's booth, is a "listening and spoken language" school. Listening and speaking were, I thought, obvious choices for Julia. She has ample residual hearing. Hearing aids work well. It was a simple equation.

Our tour of the DePaul School revealed classroom teachers using various strategies to train the kids to rely exclusively on spoken language. They held shields in front of their mouths to prevent lip reading and would not use gestures to support understanding. The institution produced results in the form of kids with varying levels of hearing loss that are fully verbal. I didn't really think much of the methods at the time. I attended a parent support group at DePaul even though Julia wasn't placed there. DePaul is affiliated with AG Bell, so I joined that as well.

In 2010, I won a sponsorship from Prilosec OTC to partially fund a trip to the AG Bell biennial conference in Orlando, FL. Tim, Julia, and I traveled to the Hilton Bonnet Creek where I was registered for the conference, Julia would attend the kid program, and Tim had an appointment with the lazy river. This was a fabulous plan. On paper.

Julia did not like the kid program one bit. Trained, supportive adults experienced in the care of kids with hearing loss took her to a farm where she milked a cow and to SeaWorld where she watched a dolphin show. Every day was filled with wonderful Orlando entertainment.

Julia wanted Mommy to see the dolphin with her. We heard about "that time you sent me to that thing in Orlando by myself" for years! In a bad way.

The Hilton Bonnet Creek in Orlando is one of the most over-priced establishments I've encountered. It is within shuttling distance of Disney World and I would have thought it would be more family-friendly. Then we paid $8 for Julia to have a cup of milk with her night snack.

The hotel milk debacle prompted Tim to rent a bicycle and ride seven miles round trip to obtain bottled water and a half gallon of milk. I think he did this because though the lazy river was beautiful, the rafts had to be rented. So, his planned relaxing flotation time was without flotation.

That left me to long days of workshops in an over air-conditioned hotel knowing full well my family was miserable. Also, I'm not a very social person. There were useful workshops, but most were geared toward professionals rather than parents. Even with these various challenges, the conference provided some helpful tips and lots of blog post material.

Thoughts on the AG Bell Session: Humor

A Magic Ear Kids blog post from July 18, 2010:

Julia learned a new joke while we were in Florida. It's a knock knock joke and I've explained it to her. I'm not entirely sure she knows why it's funny.

Knock knock.
Who's there?
Owls.
Owls who?
You're right, owls do say hoo!

This has momentarily replaced the knock knock joke punchlines, "orange you glad I didn't say banana" and "lettuce in it's cold outside." If you've spent any time with a kid lately, I'm sure you know those ones.

Since we're already spending hours answering knock

knocks and decoding inane Popsicle stick jokes, the concurrent session on humor as an auditory-verbal tool really peaked my interest. I'm not an auditory-verbal therapist and my daughter has never been specifically taught in that type of environment. My perspective is just that of a Mom that wants to help her little girl's emerging sense of comedy.

In the hour-long session, I discovered a lot of work we can be doing to understand the puns that grace our Popsicle sticks. The presenter suggested breaking riddles into two parts and having the child tell everything they know about each part.

One of her examples was: What kind of parties do lambs like?

The adult and the child can talk about all the different kinds of parties there are: birthday parties, slumber parties, graduation parties. Then everything you know about lambs: they're also called sheep, they go baa, they have wool.

Then you're supposed to help the kid make a guess at the riddle. The answer: A sheep over.

This is a great thinking and listening exercise. It's also more fun that other kinds of "work" that kids are asked to do. I wrote a bunch of silly kid jokes in my notebook.

My next step is to get a book of jokes from the library. Julia has been wanting one. Now I'm somewhat professionally trained to work through it with her. She'll soon be the Last Comic Standing, I'm sure.

***

Stress and the Hard of Hearing Child

A Magic Ear Kids blog post from August 15, 2010:

The AG Bell session, **I Can't, I Won't, I Don't Want To,** seemed like it might offer some help for problems we have at home. It's tough to distinguish whether the type of childhood anxiety we experience here on a day to day basis is from hearing loss or perhaps just the manifestation of my DNA. I was a high stress kid. Julia has moments. Either way, the stress is there.

I detect stress in her on days when she's been playing with her peers without me. I try not to seem overly self-important here, but I do mom things that help her a great deal. I use those deep knee bends to get to her level and speak at a rate that is easy to understand. I give her plenty of time to talk. I listen carefully to what she says. I worry that I've created an alternate reality where communication is different than it will be during those full days of kindergarten.

I worry because I can tell when she's spent a whole day with kids. Her emotions are on a hair trigger. She seems more tired. She's more apt to cry at a transition time or jump to a conclusion that leads to a meltdown. She has stress.

So, I was tuned in to this subject in Orlando. I was hopeful that there would be answers. As with so many parenting things, there are no absolutes.

The workshop pointed out that the difference between detection and understanding. We may think our child is doing well because they detect a conversation. They may not be fully understanding the dialog. For this we are to give them "communication repair strategies." An example would be to have the child indicate, "I don't understand" or to have them ask for clarification.

Two months after taking in this information, I've yet to put any "communication repair strategies" into practice. I sometimes ask, "Did you understand? Did you hear?" I'm at a loss as to transferring this to a self-advocacy goal. I don't know how to make her ask for clarification.

The presenters also suggested "listening breaks." They mentioned some kids that like to take their amplification off for a few hours after school. They said a child might benefit from quiet time in a small space where they can just relax.

The best I've done is to incorporate Julia's favorite play, our one on one time with Barbie dolls, into most days. She has no interest in removing her hearing aids. She has no interest in ever being alone. She never wants to be quiet herself and would always engage me in conversation. I do find that a good hour of playing with her and her dolls does relax her. So, we just have weird listening breaks.

Finally, they discussed previewing and pre-teaching as stress reducing tools. I've been working on this in different situations. We talk through who is going to be at an event and what we'll do. I've also tried to give her some coping strategies for when she feels angry or sad. We talk about the appropriate responses.

All of these tactics are trial and error endeavors for each child. I've already crossed those completely quiet listening breaks off my list. I'm still not finding a substantial improvement with the other stuff.

I'm left to wonder if I'm capable of teaching someone to manage stress. I can barely handle my own.

***

AG Bell Session: Working Memory

A Magic Ear Kids blog post from August 1, 2010:

While I was waiting for an AG Bell session on social media to begin, I overheard some people talking about the session next door. It had drawn a standing-room-only crowd. No wonder there were only a handful of people assembled to talk about twittering.

The next day, people were still abuzz with that popular session. It was about "working memory." Working memory is the ability to manipulate and access information in short-term memory. The implication is that children with hearing loss have difficulties with their working memory.

A second working memory session by a different professional was offered the next day. I attended with a smaller crowd, presumably the overflow that couldn't fit in the first one. A study was presented where typically hearing children and children with varying levels of hearing loss were put through a program to increase their working memory. Their language skills were tested before and after. Improved working memory is thought to spur language development.

The researcher found what she deemed to be statistically significant improvement in the kids with hearing loss. The kids improved their language skills by spending time on a touch screen computer duplicating patterns of flashing colors. Remembering patterns enhances working memory. It is thought that the benefits disappear as soon as the practice ends.

The experts attempted to draw a huge distinction between short-term memory and working memory. They theorized that kids with hearing loss spend a lot of energy to understand speech and have less brain power left for working memory. The miserably boring task of replicating these flashing color patterns could help.

The concept is interesting, but there isn't any fix for use in the home yet. The session served to bring me up to speed on the buzz words. It can be difficult in our house learning new friends' names and learning new words. I don't know if it's a working memory problem or not, but it's interesting to learn about this research.

***

The conference wasn't a waste by any means, but I wouldn't go to another one. A photo taken while I was dropping Julia off for the children's program has made its way into the AG Bell magazine *Volta Voices* as well as local AG Bell chapter advertising. As our needs evolved, it became apparent that we need gesture and probably should learn ASL. Though it's AG Bell's position that they support our right to choose any methodology, I don't get that vibe from them. It's more of a speak or die atmosphere.

After the conference, we spent a day at the Magic Kingdom. We headed home knowing that we won't do Orlando in June again. It's just too hot even for conferring with Mickey Mouse.

American Society for Deaf Children

The other side of the aisle from the DePaul/AG Bell no visual support method is the American Society for Deaf Children (ASDC). The affiliated school in our area, the Western Pennsylvania School for the Deaf (WPSD), offers a total communication program.

WPSD teaches children who are deaf and hard of hearing to communicate using sign language as well as auditory oral techniques. I never had occasion to visit WPSD, but I was a member of ASDC.

Though the two organizations, AG Bell and ASDC, bear no ill will toward each other on a national level, there is deep division among regular people. One attendee at a parent support group told a tale of her children being asked to leave DePaul because she used ASL to tell them goodbye as they were getting out of the car. I don't know if that's true or not, but the story was just the tip of a deep, cold iceberg that divides the hearing loss community as surely as a discussion about whether or not to capitalize the "d" in "deaf." The parent promptly transferred her children from DePaul to WPSD where they were able to sign freely.

It is my understanding that capital "D" "Deaf" refers to a community that identifies as culturally Deaf with their own language (ASL here in America) and customs. A person with hearing loss might say they are little "d" "deaf." That is basically just another way of indicating they have hearing loss and gives no indication of their attitude toward communication mode.

I was once educated by a Deaf man communicating via a sign language interpreter that Alexander Graham Bell himself was the very worst human ever to have walked the earth. The man also had a long diatribe about the existence of hearing aids and cochlear implants. He felt those technologies implied he was broken and he was most certainly not. The man was not affiliated with any organization to my knowledge and this interaction happened at an event that was not sponsored by either group.

It presents a marked difficulty to a parent of a child that wears hearing aids to be told that you're really just trying to force your child to be like you, i.e. "hearing" when God made them Deaf. That certainly hadn't been my thought process. Not getting the hearing aids was never an option.

I did once talk to a grandmother that explained their cochlear implant decision by saying, "everyone in the family can hear and talk. Why would we all learn another language just for one person? We got him a cochlear implant, so he can hear and talk too."

Her attitude didn't sit well with me, but she was being honest. And if I'm being honest, given the choice between hearing aids and speech therapy or eschewing technology and learning ASL, I'd have chosen the hearing aids. Our family might someday become fluent in sign language, but not many in the rest of the world will.

These debates simmer under the surface of the support groups and still, from my perspective, define the missions of each association. Learning about these two options made me long for another choice, but for a while, I was left to create my own hybrid and existed somewhere between the two worlds.

THIS ONE'S ALL ABOUT A TURD

A Magic Ear Kids blog post from March 5, 2010:

After finishing up an IEP meeting, I asked Julia if she needed to go to the bathroom before we headed home. She thought that was a good idea. We headed off to the elementary school bathroom.

We were in the fifth-grade wing of the building. A few 12-year-old girls were in and out during our time in the toilet. They got to hear a wonderful conversation.

"A turd just fell outta my bum, mama. A turd!"
"Shouldn't you wipe then?" I asked.
"No."

There was some more back and forth on this issue. She was insistent that a bodily function had just occurred but lives in some alternate reality where no further action was required. I was aware we had an audience and wanted to go home. I let it slide and mused that my mother of the year certificate was probably in the mail as we walked back to the meeting room.

When we got back, Julia's teacher of the deaf asked,

"Did you find the bathroom Julia?"

There was no response. The child was clearly tired.

"Are you just pooped?" was her next question.
My daughter exclaimed, "a little turd fell out!"

At this point the teacher got down to Julia's level. I was mortified that this was the moment when another adult had to explain to my child that it is inappropriate to announce what just happened in the bathroom in such detail.

"It's an expression," the teacher told her. "Pooped means you feel tired!"

It may not have been the best time to introduce that particular expression. "Are you pooped?" and "did you poop?" are rather close phrases. Combined with the proximity to an actual bathroom trip, this probably motivated the unabashed disclosure. Or it could be that Julia was just really hung up on that turd.

Apparently, the teacher and another attendee of our IEP meeting had just been having some sort of conversation about the difficulties children with hearing loss face. "This is a perfect example," the teacher exclaimed as I turned fifteen shades of red. "This is perfect for your blog!"

Maybe. If you're the sort of person that will blog about a turd. Fortunately for you, I am.

A MOM WITH LARYNGITIS AND A KID WITH HEARING LOSS

A Magic Ear Kids blog post from March 19, 2010:

The whole family came down with a mild cold this week. Julia had it first. By the time Tim got it I was pretty sure the thing was unavoidable. I'm about four days in now.

Sinus headaches, joint pain, and a runny nose are annoying enough when you're chasing an energetic youngster around. I had all that and I lost my voice. I spent the day yesterday ranging from decreased volume and squeaking to nothing but a faint whisper.

Julia couldn't hear me.

I'm used to repeating myself and talking louder than normal. I even spell things sometimes which amazes me because a preschooler shouldn't be helped by that kind of thing. I found myself trapped with no extra volume and no vocal stamina to repeat each phrase until she got it.

I explained the situation several times. She didn't get it.

I think it was the most miserable day we've had together since the stress-induced tantrums just after she turned four. She didn't kick or bite me, but she seemed injured because I couldn't hold up my end of the conversation. That hurts worse than being bitten. By late afternoon she was fed up with me.

Dad had to read the nighttime stories and Julia said her own prayers. "Help Mommy get over her cold," she said.

Please do.

SELF-ADVOCACY AMUSEMENTS

A Magic Ear Kids blog post from April 11, 2010:

It was really hot last week, and the two sisters next door were in their bathing suits to jump on the trampoline while it was being sprayed with a hose. Julia adores this trampoline and barges in on it at every opportunity. This day, she couldn't because her hearing aids can't get wet.

We're new to the neighborhood and these "will you play with me?" conversations are a bit awkward. Julia went up to the youngest of the neighbors and said hello.

"I can't go on there with the water. I can't get my hair wet," Julia told her.
The other little girl was swaying shyly.
"I wear magic ears," Julia continued.

At this point, I prompted Julia to show the girls her hearing aids since they probably have no idea what she was talking about.

Julia lifted her hair and said, "These are my magic ears.

They help me hear. Without them I can't hear very well. You have to talk really loud. Look, these are my earrings, and these are my magic ears. Can you tell the difference? It's very confusing."

She also pointed out that she was wearing aqua socks and it is okay if they get wet.

Self-advocacy will be a goal of ours for quite some time. Julia has to be able to position herself to hear in the classroom and social settings. She needs to be able to explain her hearing aids to her peers. My husband and I felt reassured listening to this conversation. She advocates for herself pretty well already!

MOTIVATING HEARING AID INDEPENDENCE

A Magic Ear Kids blog post from May 2, 2010:

I decided Julia should learn to put her hearing aids in on her own. We'd tried it just prior to getting new ear molds. She was doing okay then. Then the new sparkly ones were too snug and sticky for her to get in on her own.

Months later, she turned five. Her ears have grown just enough to allow easy ear mold insertion.

I tied her hair up and gave her a speech about the red dot showing which one is for her right ear. I handed her the hearing aid and put her in front of a mirror. I explained which part of the mold lines up with which part of her ear. I demonstrated. I coached.

"I can't do it," she said.

She'd barely tried, essentially smashing her hearing aid at her ear in a haphazard fashion.

"You're not trying," I said calmly.

We were about 20 minutes into a task that I could do for her in 20 seconds.

"If you can't learn to do this on your own," I told her, "you're not going to be allowed to go on a slumber party with your cousin."

"I can do it!" she shouted.

Those hearing aids were in and turned on in a couple of minutes. Each following attempt was successful and met with an excited girl screeching, "Mommy, I got to the point! I can go on a slumber party!"

The slumber party is scheduled for May 21st. She can do anything. All it takes is proper motivation.

HIDE AND SEEK WITH HEARING AIDS

A Magic Ear Kids blog post from May 9, 2010:

Julia has been learning to insert her hearing aids in her own little ears. It was going well. Then without even thinking anything of it, I handed her both hearing aids and went downstairs to make dinner.

Julia had just spent an hour in our big bathtub pretend swimming. Bathing suit, snorkel, diving rings, and goggles; she had the whole deal. Afterward, I had dried her hair and tied it up while she was wrapped in a towel. When I left her, she was diligently working on inserting her right aid.

She was supposed to finish with the hearing aids and then go put on clothing. Thirty minutes passed as I worked on assembling tacos and making some Rice-a-roni. I was enjoying the time as I thought she was entertaining herself.

Then I heard a soft voice, “Mommy, I can’t find my magic ear.”

I abandoned the Rice-a-roni to find a strangely dressed child wearing one hearing aid. She lost a hearing aid and just wandered off to get dressed. Ever think of looking for it before you go put on your Little Mermaid dress?

"I can't find the other one," she says.
"Where is it?" I wanted to know. I guess that was a dumb question. She didn't know where it was.

I started the sort of frenzied search that never allows a person to find anything. All the while I'm bombarding her with questions in a raised, unhappy voice. She just sat on my cedar chest in the same place I left her when she still had two hearing aids. She seemed unaffected by the drama that was playing out.

All kinds of thoughts went through my mind: toilet, chewing by dog. I wondered if she hid it on purpose. I tried to collect myself and sat down with her.

"Tell me exactly what happened," I told her. "Start with what happened right after you finished putting the first one in."
"I took the other one," she said while taking a deep breath, "and I threw it up in the air. I'm very afraid it's on the ceiling fan."

For crap's sake. If you can imagine, I really do pseudo swear even in my own mind. I headed downstairs to call for reinforcements.

I had to flag the Dad down because he was mowing the lawn. I explained the situation to him and he immediately began searching the bedroom with me. He asked her to explain what had happened. At that moment, she began to show emotion. Mom had been flipping out for 15 minutes but suddenly having to tell Dad what happened made her feel all BAD.

"You are not ready for a slumber party," I hissed.

Then I moved the cedar chest and found the hearing aid safe and sound underneath. Lots of deep breathing later we decided as a family that she might still have her slumber party reward if she can demonstrate responsible hearing aid care in the meantime. Not throwing the things at the ceiling fan will be a good start.

CONVENTIONAL AUDIOMETRIC TEST PROCEDURES OR A "BIG GIRL" BOOTH TEST

A Magic Ear Kids blog post from June 13, 2010:

At the end of May, Julia returned to the audiologist. It had been only three months since the last test. She's on a more frequent schedule because her middle frequencies have gotten a bit worse.

The booth hasn't been a great thing to witness in the past few appointments. Julia had been difficult to keep on task and didn't seem too interested in feeding elephants, monkeys, dogs and rabbits as part of her conditioned response to hearing a sound.

Our audiologist decided for the most recent test that Julia was ready for "conventional audiometric test procedures." What a difference! I think Jules relished hearing the audiologist throughout the testing.

She had to repeat words for the word recognition test rather than pointing at pictures. She shouted her responses so loud I wished I had ear plugs. Julia proudly pronounced every sound in each word.

Conventional procedures call for the child to raise their hand after hearing each sound. Julia was quite enthusiastic with this one as well. She did an all-around outstanding job.

Last night, I got the two-page written report titled: Audiology Evaluation. It included a new audiogram and a detailed description of the tests and results. It didn't mention how the audiologist turned down her headphones to keep from having her own eardrums injured by the enthusiasm of my young child. It left out how proud she was to raise her hand as soon as she heard each "whistle."

Thankfully this post will round out the report because those were details too precious to forget.

KINDERGARTEN HERE WE COME

Kindergarten was a huge deadline for us from the moment Julia's hearing loss was diagnosed. We only thought about ears in our house and the point of our existence was to have them ready for school. Julia's speech was caught up to her typically hearing peers by her fourth birthday. We spent the extra year and a half working on the rest of the kindergarten readiness goals.

Our district has a full-day kindergarten program. Julia was going to go from full days at home with me to seven-hour stints away from home. This was toughest on me and I would have done anything to stop the clock in that last summer before the start of school.

My fears ranged from her having difficulty hearing with everything working properly to equipment malfunctions to another kid eating one of her hearing aids. I didn't even have the energy to worry about someone teasing her. My mind was completely occupied by the horrors that might befall her equipment.

We were able to meet the teacher ahead of time. She had a degree in special education and was unfazed by the FM system. The school district had chosen her for Julia because she was one of the few teachers that used a built-in sound field system in her classroom every day no matter what. The added support of the sound field was a comfort and the teacher was already used to wearing a microphone.

By the time Julia got on the bus, I had only to worry about what I was going to do all day. I was alone, but she was in good hands. I might have had unnecessary anxiety over our preparedness, but prepared she was. We looked forward to a successful school career knowing we'd done all we could do to be ready for it.

Classroom strategies for mild/moderate hearing loss

A Magic Ear Kids blog post from March 28, 2010:

IEP time came for us again in February. Having moved from one county to another and then back again, it seems like a lot of meetings for one little kid. Now we're in our forever home and have written the all-important IEP that will be used for her transition to kindergarten.

There are only two goals this time. Speech has been conquered and now the task is to make sure she continues to grow as a listener. The first goal is to maintain her skills. The second is about following directions. This IEP will hopefully keep her from falling behind because of her hearing loss.

Julia's Teacher of the Deaf and Hard of Hearing wrote a great list of strategies needed to achieve these goals.

They are:

- Minimize background noise
- Use preferential seating in a large group with appropriate access to peers and teacher
- In small groups and one-on-one situations seat Julia in front of or next to the speaker
- Utilize auditory sandwich techniques (presenting information verbally, pausing to wait for a response, giving a visual clue, then repeating verbal information)
- Provide extra time for processing
- Provide acoustic highlighting techniques to enhance the audibility of spoken language (whispering or emphasizing a specific pitch)
- Use rephrasing and repetition to supplement verbal instruction
- Model appropriate language
- Expand and extend Julia's spontaneous utterances
- Speak at normal conversational levels at close range
- Identify who is speaking and repeat/paraphrase information stated by her peers
- Use a varied vocabulary with Julia to convey a variety of concepts
- Give breaks from listening
- Encourage Julia to use clarification as needed and begin to self-advocate
- Implement the proper use of an FM system

We've come so far, but there's still a lot to be done. Like me, Julia has significant difficulty understanding other kids. Most recently she complained that with her FM she could only hear her dance teacher and not her friends. We're continuing to learn and adapt as a family with the above list of strategies as our guide.

Kindergarten Accommodations

A Magic Ear Kids blog post from September 12, 2010:

Julia has finished her first two weeks of kindergarten. She loves it! So far everything has been going smoothly.

Julia wears two Phonak eXtra 311 behind-the-ear hearing aids. The school has purchased a Phonak Inspiro FM system for her use during the school day. I was impressed with the system, compared to the Phonak EasyLink we have at home. The Inspiro has a nifty test for the teacher to make sure the microphone is in the correct position. It requires the teacher to read a sentence and shows a smiley face on the display if it is correctly positioned. We've had trouble with microphone placement during the preschool years. Hopefully we won't have any issues now.

Each morning when Julia gets into her class, she takes her hearing aids out and puts the FM receivers on by herself. The boots go back and forth between school and home, but the receivers have to stay at the school. I was a bit worried about this part. Thankfully, Julia has really mastered taking her aids out and putting them in. I'm still making sure her hair is pulled back to keep things as simple as possible.

Three times a week Julia is pulled out of the classroom to work for 30 minutes with her hearing support teacher. They are working on self-advocacy goals, lip reading, and caring for the hearing aids. The hearing support teacher will also help the classroom teacher to implement the classroom strategies in the IEP.

Starting kindergarten has been a great experience. We got to meet Julia's teacher and see her classroom for the first time at the beginning of summer. Knowing the teachers ahead of time helped us when we were preparing for the big first day of school. Here's hoping the rest of the year goes just as well as the beginning!

Staying in the elementary school loop

A Magic Ear Kids blog post from November 21, 2010:

Julia quickly tires of my after-school questions. I have to wait for things to come out. It requires patience and restraint on my part.

In the first weeks I wanted her to report on the faculty's use of her FM system. Are they using it? Does it help her?

Julia was patient with me, but didn't reveal many details on the subject. I was almost relieved the morning I left the FM boots off of her hearing aids. At least the teacher noticed. That means she uses it!

Since consciously sabotaging equipment isn't a great plan, I've found a better way to stay in the loop during these elementary school years.

I spy.

I went deep under cover during my first spy mission as a parent-teacher group volunteer. I had to pack some boxes to clean up after the book fair, but the information I gathered in the school lobby was quite valuable.

A guy from our church was in the school to talk to the kids about trees. They took a walk around the playground to collect leaves. I took the opportunity to say "hello."

"I had Julia in my group yesterday," he told me. "They put the microphone on me and everything."

This is good. I spied, and they passed!

I feel confident the school has adopted the assistive technology as a part of the daily routine. I'm happy. It's nice knowing what's going on, even if I have to occasionally do a little heavy lifting.

Fly on the wall with feelings

A Magic Ear Kids blog post from December 12, 2010:

During my two weeks of sickness, I assembled enough energy to volunteer for a day at Julia's school. I loaded my pockets with tissues and cough drops. Soon I found myself lost in a chorus of coughing and sniffling. I didn't need to worry about standing out in the crowd.

It was Thanksgiving Eve and the kindergarten wing

was filled with parent helpers. The rare full day volunteer opportunity found us making tee-pees out of tortillas and apple turkeys. Kindergarten teachers are like craft ninjas, they fashioned a turkey call out of a plastic cup, some string and a sponge.

I helped and watched my daughter navigate a school day.

She stood with her class to recite the Pledge of Allegiance and was called aside to put on her FM receivers. I cringed and felt a tinge of sadness. She went to the far side of the classroom and pulled her squealing hearing aids out. In a moment she had one receiver lined up. The kindergarten teacher helped her snap it in place. By the end of the Pledge, the FM was up and running.

After each activity, the kids went to a different room for another teacher's activity. Julia transported the FM transmitter. She clipped it to her own waistband and attached the microphone to her collar. She looked like a little mini-teacher.

Each of the kindergarten teachers knew all about the FM system. They positioned it appropriately and tested to make sure it was working. In a flurry of instructions these teachers would say, "Julia." Jules would jump or suddenly turn around. It was comical in a slightly painful way.

By the end of the day, I managed to replace my sadness with pride. Here is a little girl that fully understands the accommodations offered to give her full access to sound. She handles her hearing aids and the FM system with confidence. She takes this all as just a part of her day. She doesn't envy the other kids. She even enjoys having that little microphone. She'll sing herself a song into it when she has a chance.

She's an inspiration. Though I'm sure it won't always be so easy for her, she's got this kindergarten thing locked down. It helps that the staff at her school is pretty extraordinary too.

THE KINDERGARTEN MELTDOWN

Another parent once told me that the hearing loss journey isn't like climbing a mountain, it's like being stuck on a bicycle wheel. You go up and up, struggling to a plateau and then suddenly cruise down with no resistance. Eventually, you have to go up again because it's a wheel and that's what wheels do.

Though our experience hasn't been all that dramatic, there have been pinch points. Moments in our family history that squeeze and make me uncomfortable. Moments of indecision and self-doubt. Moments of despair.

Kindergarten was a huge milestone for hearing support, self-advocacy, and independence. It required me to let go and trust other adults with expensive equipment. It forced me to put the very sweetest little girl in the world on a big yellow bus and send her away for a whole day.

She went and really did flourish for three quarters of her kindergarten year. By Thanksgiving I'd reassured myself of the competency of the school staff by volunteering at every opportunity. With life cruising on that downhill part of the hearing loss wheel, I applied to be a substitute special education paraprofessional and reentered the workforce. Some days I was in Julia's building. Other days I worked an earlier schedule at the high school or middle school, dropping Julia at daycare to have breakfast and get on the bus.

By spring, kindergarteners were prepping for the annual Mother's Day program. Tim was traveling often for work and I was dropping Julia at the daycare every morning for a three-week stint subbing for a high school para that was having back surgery. Then the wonderful kindergarten teacher with a special education degree that used the sound field no matter what went on maternity leave.

And our world fell apart.

The substitute kindergarten teacher was a young man, probably a recent college grad, with a palpable distain for children. Julia began to cry every day. She didn't want to go to school anymore.

We enlisted the help of the school guidance counselor and tried to talk through the many objections Julia had developed to the school day she once loved. There was no solution. She was clearly miserable.

Our troubles came to a head one night when she burst into tears about an art project she'd been working on at school.

"I can't get the circles right," she choked through her tears. "They're all lumpy."

"It doesn't matter if the circles are perfectly smooth circles," I told her. "You know there's no right or wrong when it comes to making art. Elmo says that."

Not even Elmo could save us.

We muddled through that spring as a family. The week before Mother's Day we assembled in the school's multipurpose room for the carefully prepared program. The kids sang a long set of songs about mothers, *You Are My Sunshine*, and other adorable classics. All around me there were parents with prideful eyes glistening with tears. It was moving to be sure.

I felt sick that evening. Absolutely sick. Up on the stage, there was my pride and joy, trying to sing, trying to make something "special" and "perfect" for mommy. She couldn't remember the words.

I knew in that moment that our whole IEP had failed. It was meant to give extra support for emerging skills and it left her in daily practice with no reinforcement for complicated lyrics that she wasn't able to master. Those songs should have been sent home for extra practice, but they were a "surprise for mommy."

That week she brought home the offending art project. It was Eric Carle's *Very Hungry Caterpillar* and the circles were really quite circular.

"This is so good," I told her.

Tear filled eyes indicated that it just wasn't good enough.

The kindergarten meltdown led to additional line items in the IEP. More than anything, it made me glad for the ever-increasing communication abilities my daughter gained day by day. Things she couldn't express when she was six became easier for her to convey over time. Our conversations about school eventually uncovered the art teacher's insistence that every kid's work must look as close to her example as possible. It really wasn't an art class, but a complex step by step copying workroom. The process didn't jibe with Julia's creative leanings and the teacher never chose a single piece of her work for the many display windows in the school.

It was frustrating for a creative young girl. Art class continued to be a problem until we were able to have more grown up conversations about the nature of artistic expression and the value of these paint by number type projects. It was a lesson to me as a parent that problems aren't resolved in the elementary years by sending a note to teacher that says, "let my daughter make her caterpillar as lumpy as she wants." Advocacy becomes about working with your child to help them identify their needs and make confident requests of the adults around them.

It's more difficult than firing off notes, but hopefully it will pay off in the future.

***

Future IEP notes

A Magic Ear Kids blog post from February 13, 2011:

Working as a special education paraprofessional in our local school district has given me lots of exposure to

Julia's future educational environment. I've worked in different classrooms in first through fifth grade. I've spent time in the middle school. Currently, I'm doing a stint in high school.

The grade school teachers ask for students to get up and answer math questions. The little children give correct answers while facing the white board in barely audible voices. This is going to be a problem.

An assembly turned boy versus girl shouting match got really loud. Several special needs kids were pulled into the hallway to escape the sound of competitive screaming/shrieking. This is going to be a problem.

High school students are required to swim as part of gym class. I learned that kids with an IEP can opt out of this requirement. Good to know.

So, I have a page in my trusty notebook dedicated to "ideas for future IEPs." For next year we'll talk about tennis balls on chair legs, the sound field and personal FM. I'll inquire about getting a Mic for those student teachers to help clarify their shy white board mumblings. I'll ask that Julia have the option to remove herself from any assemblage of shrieking kids or at least have someone knowledgeable enough to remind her of her hearing aid volume control.

I feel informed and prepared from my time spent subbing. Come IEP time I'll be prepared with my notebook. There's stuff in there for years to come.

DEALING WITH THE PEOPLE THAT ARE NEVER GONNA GET IT

Hearing loss and the resulting IEP have given Julia the very best educational experience a parent could want. She's always been in classrooms with patient, experienced teachers. As much as is possible, the adults in her life have made learning easier on her. At least, the playing field has been kept close to what typically hearing children are using.

It can't be avoided that there are people in the world that simply aren't capable of understanding hearing loss. I'd be willing to bet they have difficulty with the nuances of other conditions as well, but my experience is exclusive to hearing.

Whenever possible, we try first to educate the uninitiated about Julia's specific hearing loss. She's blessed to have enough residual hearing to make out loud speech at close range without her hearing aids. Hearing loss has made swimming lessons difficult, but not impossible. Two out of three swim instructors have been able to make it work.

All but a couple of teachers have adjusted to using the

FM system even if they can't understand why it's necessary.

From time to time, I find myself explaining hearing loss and walking away with the distinct impression I've made no positive impact whatsoever on the other person's understanding. As long as they're doing what's required of them for my child, they can be confused. The accommodations are the important bit. We can work on educating the masses later.

Swim class

A Magic Ear Kids blog post from July 12, 2011:

For the past two summers, I've thought about enrolling Julia in a swimming class. She is a true water baby, a fearless, underwater mermaid type.

Swimming is complicated. We've learned a bit of ASL and I talk pretty loud right in her ear. We get by together at the pool.

Group instruction with Julia unaided seemed pointless at best. Thinking that someone must have encountered this problem before, I talked to people at the Western Pennsylvania School for the Deaf. They had no advice.

Finally, friends of ours told us about a fantastic swim class offered by a local woman in her backyard pool. I signed Julia up. Then I had the requisite two nights of anxiety dreams while anticipating the start of class.

The program is fabulous, but the setting still presents many challenges. One of the instructors, a teenage boy, turns his voice off and makes exaggerated lip movements. He also attempts to pantomime. I told him that he can just talk loud at close range. He seems to think that's weirder than what he's been doing. Eventually, I plopped myself at the side of the pool to keep Julia from floating into the deep end while simultaneously directing her to stay above the water while they're demonstrating new strokes. I repeated some of the directions loudly into her ears.

I signed "pay attention" a lot.

I felt tired when the class ended.

The effort seems to be paying off. There seems to be some structure being added to her movements. She taught her instructors how to sign "kick." Surely, by the end of class they'll also pick up "wait" and "pay attention."

Everyone is learning and I'm proud of us. Truly, anything is possible.

An Idiot's Guide to Ear Problems

A Magic Ear Kids blog post from July 13, 2012:

A real breakthrough has been made this week in our child's swimming ability. Monday was the first day of swim class. The same swim class Julia took last summer complete with the same three instructors.

I've been sitting, relaxing even, poolside, while two out of three instructors repeat the instructions at close range. They check to make sure Julia knows what she should do. Julia is paying attention without any prompting. Her determination and the instructors' accommodations have made all the difference. After three lessons, Julia figured out how to swim on top of the water. She coordinates her little arms and turns her head to the side. It's slow, but steady, and close to accurate.

I am thrilled.

There's still that third instructor though. Last year, I figured him for a teenager. Maybe he's in college. Either way, he doesn't get it.

On Monday, Julia interacted only with the two accommodating instructors. I thought this might have been by design. The boy has lots of other kids to work with.

Shortly into the lesson on Tuesday, he came for Julia. "YOU. GO. DO IT!" he barked.

By that he meant, "please float on your front for five seconds and then flip on to your back and float for five seconds."

Julia looked at him quizzically and thrashed around in the water. He attempted some crude pantomime. More thrashing. The boy eventually grabbed her by the arm and moved her back into the waiting area.

She was back with the preferred teachers for a few skills and then as luck would have it, again with the boy. This time he indicated her turn with a forceful jab of his finger.

In three steps I was hovering over him, "Excuse me, she really needs you to repeat the instructions at close range. That pancake flip you took her for last time didn't go well because the communication wasn't there. The other two instructors have been having success making sure she knows what to do before they take her. You need to explain it to her again or maybe just let the other teachers take her. That would be fine too."

I turned back toward my chair. I'd said my piece. It wasn't really a conversation, but then I heard him talking.

"I know," he said. I turned around. "We've had kids before with cochlear implants."
"She doesn't have a cochlear implant," I said, possibly cutting him off. "It's not the same thing."
"Yeah," he shrugged. "I get it. She has an ear problem."

And you have an idiot problem.

Thankfully, his boss, one of the two preferred instructors, interceded and informed the boy that he should just repeat the directions.

It's been a good opportunity for Julia to work on her self-advocacy skills. "Don't go unless you know what you're supposed to do," I told her after class. Tim suggested we teach her to say, "Hey (insert alternate name for a donkey), I didn't hear you!"

That may be a little much.

By this afternoon, the boy was doing better during the few times he instructed Julia. It seems like Julia is much less inclined to guess at what she should do. She objects when she doesn't understand. It helps that she's getting the hang of her swim strokes. And that two of the instructors are really going above and beyond. Perhaps Meatloaf was right, "two out of three ain't bad."

Parking Lot Revelations

A Magic Ear Kids blog post from October 23, 2012:

Our community loves parades. It must because twice per year more than half of us march down the street throwing candy at the few people that aren't in the event themselves. Julia also loves a parade. More than anything, she loves being in the parade.

In mid-September we marched in our third parade since living here. It takes a long time prepping for one of these deals. You must arrive an hour before it starts. You must stand in the parking lot, shifting from foot to foot, conversing with the other mothers, directing your child not to eat the candy that they're so excited to throw in the street. You must love your child. You would not choose to do this for any other reason.

This year, Julia's second grade class (taught by Mrs. L) has three girls that are also in her Brownie troop. It provided a bit more fodder for the pre-parade conversation. We talked about which boys our daughters mention and what they play at recess.

Then the other mom, we'll call her Inquisitive Mom, asked, "So Mrs. L wears that thing around her neck. What's that thing she wears around her neck?"

"Oh, she has a sound field in her classroom. It amplifies her voice using the four speakers in the classroom," I say.

"But Julia doesn't need that, does she? Is it for Julia?" probes the Inquisitive Mom.

Suddenly, I feel defensive and weird. "The sound field isn't specifically for Julia," I sputter. "Mrs. L has always used it. It's hooked up so that Julia's FM works with it. Mrs. L wears one microphone and it goes into the speakers and Julia's hearing aids."

"But she doesn't need that does she? I mean you wouldn't even know there's anything... with her. You can't tell," says Inquisitive Mom.

"She could probably get by without it," I say.
Why did I just say that?
"What it does for her is it reduces the listening distance," *I'm still talking.*

This woman has no idea what I'm saying and all she's going to remember is that we make the teacher wear an unnecessary microphone because it gives us pleasure to make people do our bidding.

"Instead of being ten feet away from Julia, the FM

makes it like the teacher is right next to her talking. It helps a lot when they're learning new vocabulary and when Julia needs to discriminate between similar sounds."

I used way too many big words.

Another mom joins the conversation, agreeing that Julia shows no signs of needing any special accommodations. It's a backhanded compliment. I nod and say, "yes, she does very well."

I mention that Julia's first grade teacher always used a sound field, even before Julia was in her class. I tell them that both teachers find that it really helps all of the kids. The students have better behavior and attend well to their lessons. I tell them that Julia did better when using the sound field and the FM as opposed to personal FM only. The moms agree. "You gotta do what works."

The conversation turns and eventually the parade blissfully ends.

A week later, Julia came home from school filled with facts about the classroom butterflies that had just emerged from their cocoons.

"Do you know what a butterfly mouth is called, Mommy?"
"No."
"It's a KAboscis!"
"Wow," I laugh. "That's a funny word."

For an entire weekend, Mom, Dad, and Julia made KAboscis jokes. "Shut your KAboscis," was used more than once. Julia got a new stuffed animal and named it Twinkle KAboscis.

Eventually, a paper came home from school with a diagram of butterfly parts. A butterfly mouth is called a proboscis.

She needs the FM. Even with it, strange new words are challenging.

I'm glad that my daughter has wonderful speech and holds up her end of a conversation. I'm glad random parking lot moms can't tell how much she needs her hearing aids and classroom accommodations. But I'd advise society as a whole to be careful when making judgements about what children need. There's often more to it than meets the eye.

DIBELS AND OTHER NONSENSE

A Magic Ear Kids blog post from December 11, 2012:

Second grade has been interesting. That is to say, Julia adores her teacher, loves school, and every day I think about pulling the plug on it and homeschooling her. I think that's called a dichotomy: my equally impressive, simultaneous, and completely opposing feelings that school is great and I don't want to send her there anymore.

It started with the DIBELS. "'The Dynamic Indicators of Basic Early Literacy Skills' (DIBELS) are a set of procedures and measures for assessing the acquisition of early literacy skills from kindergarten through sixth grade." Basically, it's a test given periodically to make sure students are gaining those important building blocks on the way to reading fluency.

By all accounts, Julia was doing wonderfully. One paper came home from school showing her reading comprehension on par with that of a child halfway through third grade. She was... is a fluent reader. She can understand and retell stories read to her and that she read independently. But in October, she didn't achieve benchmark on the nonsense word portion of the DIBELS.

Trouble with nonsense words seemed to snowball or at least coincide with a bunch of other less than promising findings. We discovered she couldn't decode short vowel sounds. Then I began to pick apart the mechanics of her whole process. She doesn't use phonemes but seems to read by patterns. Suddenly there are all of these holes in her emerging literacy. She has started confusing b's and d's while reading, expanding a problem that had previously been contained to just her own messy handwriting.

For a while it seemed everything was falling apart. At least one source indicated DIBELS is not a good assessment for kids with hearing loss. Should we just do away with DIBELS? But we can't let her fall behind in reading. I was starting to lose sleep over it.

Fortunately, I am in regular contact with a handful of people that have infinitely more knowledge than I do about teaching kids to read. These experts suggested visual phonics. Visual phonics pairs a hand shape/motion with each sound. There are 46 of these sounds in the English language.

I figure it's worth a try.

There was some delay in implementing visual phonics. I learned that our school district doesn't use visual phonics. They made up their own set of cues to avoid the cost of training teachers on the already developed, standardized program. Though completely baffled that there's even an option, I had to decide whether Julia should learn visual phonics (like the rest of the world) or the other thing.

We chose visual phonics.

So far, Julia has learned the cues for long and short "o". She announced afterwards that she doesn't like it and doesn't see how it's going to help.

"I never understood how this helped you remember to make an /s/ sound," I told her waving my index finger in front of my mouth like I've done so many times over the years. "But it did."

So, we're forging ahead. Julia is getting extra practice at school with those nonsense words. She's got a stack of flashcards with different syllables that she combines to make her own nonsense words. I've increased the amount of daily independent reading time she has in case it's my corrections that are messing her up when we read together. She'll learn visual phonics whether she likes it or not.

And I, always the anxious mother, will attempt to trust the public school system... and breathe.

HANDS & VOICES OF PENNSYLVANIA

A Magic Ear Kids blog post from July 1, 2012:

In 2008, I attended my first support group for parents of deaf/hard of hearing children. Julia was freshly aided but still non-verbal. Her dad and I were in full-on panic mode. The Internet did not paint a pretty picture for late-diagnosed kids.

Tears came easily in those first months, and I was eager to connect. I learned two things at the meeting:

1. My daughter wasn't "deaf enough" for me to even worry about.
2. Hearing loss is overcome exclusively through the use of intense auditory-verbal therapy.

I left feeling worse than I did going in, burdened by the guilt of my daughter's residual hearing (other kids had much less) and more anxious than ever about those years of missed speech therapy. It wasn't what I had in mind when thinking of "support."

Over the years, I met many more families and read documents promoting every methodology. I attended presentations that chastised parents for not signing because the lack of a visual support to spoken language is something akin to child abuse. Total Communication alternated between being the holy grail of Deaf Ed and a non-existent, nearly mythical misnomer. I heard research eluding to the inability of signing children to learn to speak and that they would never learn to read. All around there were pronouncements of children being "too deaf" or "not deaf enough" for one thing or the other.

In spite of these hard and fast pronouncements, happy, healthy kids were all around reading and communicating.

During this period of self-discovery, I stumbled upon Hands & Voices. "What works for your child is what makes the choice right," is their motto. Here was an organization, finally, that showed me all of the options and advocated fiercely for the rights of every deaf/hard of hearing child. Hands & Voices is a network of families supporting each other to achieve the best life for their child.

I felt a great relief as I learned more about Hands & Voices. I think it might have calmed some of my fears had I found it a few years earlier!

After bouncing between AG Bell and ASDC without feeling truly at home in either organization, Hands & Voices met my need for information and support. They reassure parents that together we can achieve positive outcomes for every child and make sure no family feels they're in this alone.

WAKING THE DEAF*

A Magic Ear Kids blog post from September 10, 2012:

Two summers ago, I attended a parents-only presentation during Pennsylvania's Great Start Conference. The doors were closed to professionals to give us all comfort and freedom talk about said professionals. I don't remember any juicy disclosures about the uninvited, but I've never forgotten one of our sidebar discussions.

"How do you wake your kid in the morning?" the presenter asked. "I don't know the answer, I seriously just want to know how you do it. Give me some ideas."

I raised my hand high. "My daughter is very sensitive to light," I replied. "I just open the blinds in the morning and fifteen minutes later she's awake."

Easy-peasy, as Julia would say.

And I knew even then that I had made a mistake. I'd jinxed it and soon, growing more mature, getting sleepier, and discovering the ever-present draw of a peaceful slumber, Julia would get over her sensitivity to light.

This summer, she slept past seven o'clock for the first time in her life. Sometimes she'd make it to 9:30, even 10:00. Sunlight was powerless to stop her.

On school mornings, I open the blinds. That serves to help me find her. Then I hug, kiss, and shake her until she's awake. Groaning she'll ask, "is it the weekend?" I sign "no" and she burrows under the covers.

Most mornings, I enlist the help of our two dogs: the fuzzy alarm clocks. They are effective past eight. Full of energy and eager for a play mate, they'll jump all over Julia, not stopping until she is upright.

Before eight, not so much. They're shih tzus. Roughly translated**, "shih tzu" means "to sleep all day." Even though they bound after me with much enthusiasm, they will very willingly curl up next to their kid for an early morning nap. She throws her arms around them and it's over. Now I have to wake a kid and two dogs.

The morning wake up is one of my favorite parts of the day. Sometimes, Julia tries to pull me under. I can score an extra hug before she really knows what's happening. Eventually, I'll have to get her an electronic device. But for now, I enjoy the morning wake up. Useless fuzzy alarm clocks and all.

*We don't normally refer to our daughter as "deaf."
**Shih Tzu does not mean "to sleep all day" although my dogs do sleep all day.

LEARNING ALL OF OUR LANGUAGE

During a heated game of Monopoly Jr., a distressed Julia, age six and a half, exclaimed, "Barn it!"

It wasn't "barn" she said exactly. It was something though that quite resembled "darn." I knew she was effectively trying out a new pseudo swear she'd half heard at school.

And there I was, squarely in the middle of a dilemma I knew was coming. Should I correct pronunciation of words I don't want her to say?

Some parents of children that are deaf or hard-of-hearing purposefully teach their children curse words. I once read a mother's blog post about equipping her deaf son with the **whole English language**. She didn't want him to be left out and, so she personally clued him in.

I knew I couldn't do that.

At some point, probably during pregnancy, I realized I don't like swearing. Arguments that they're "just words" and they only "have the power we give them" just don't cut it with me. Those words are angry and even low class. So, I say, "shoot" and "oh man" and "holy cow." If I ever slipped, I'd remind myself to be more careful. I modeled good clean speech because I don't think little kids are cute when they swear. Especially not my little kid.

But it's impractical to send a child into the world with a gaping hole in their understanding of language, so I did correct young Julia's pronunciation of "darn" that day. Then I told her we don't talk like that.

A friend with an older son that has profound hearing loss assured me that *those words* would be introduced in literature. Sure enough, even in our read aloud selections, the unsavory vocabulary words entered our home. Julia learned words that are still allowed in a radio edit.

As Julia became a proficient reader, we turned on our TV's closed captioning. Soon Tim and I were dependent on the added visual support to understand accents and slushy actor speech. Captions worked in a cyclical manner to reinforce Julia's reading skills and support listening. Before long, we looked for captions on everything.

It was the X-men that first brought the really bad words to my little girl. One evening, a closeup of Wolverine was captioned "@#$% off!" And I got to explain why we don't use "f" when we're coming up with rhymes for the word "duck."

As it turns out, from grade school on, vocabulary

grows effortlessly, even the bad parts. Books and movies quickly become more mature. Charged with choosing her own reading selections, occasionally she tells me, "I stopped reading this book because it had the f—word on every page."

That always makes me feel like a great mother!

She's also developed an affinity for comedy. It's put us into a very rich language learning environment. Now a middle schooler, she adores Tina Fey. I explain cultural references and innuendo on a regular basis. On one car ride, Julia mused that it was strange that there were so many slang words for the male reproductive organ but not the female. My resulting slang word riff made her blush. She told me then that she wished I would shelter her a little more.

"I don't want you to get caught not knowing what people are talking about," I told her.

It occurs to me that her **full** understanding has been the goal all along.

The Imperfect World of Captioning
A Magic Ear Kids blog post from December 27, 2012:

Our family likes to watch movies. Julia was completely spellbound at age three when she watched her first movie, Snow White and the Seven Dwarfs. In the past couple of years, she's matured into a bigger kid movie viewer. We watched all of the Harry Potter movies and the *Chronicles of Narnia*. We only remembered the Lord of the Rings trilogy when previews started for the new prequel, *The Hobbit.*

So, Christmas break became a *Lord of the Rings* marathon.

Quite on accident, *LOTR Fellowship of the Rings* started displaying the closed captions from the moment the DVD was inserted. Tim went for the remote to turn the captions off, but I asked him to leave them. Maybe they would help.

Watching the bigger kid movies with Julia isn't always completely enjoyable.

"What did he say?"
"What's going on?"
"What? WHAT?"

The Fellowship of the Rings was pure bliss. Julia was relaxed and didn't ask for mid-movie plot explanations. Tim and I agreed that we may not have known what was going on when we first saw the movie. Hobbits, Elves, and Orcs have tough accents. Background music crowds out the dialog. Why don't we all use closed captions?

The second movie was also a DVD with identical captions to the first. I recorded the *Return of the King* from a free preview weekend of Starz and we found those captions weren't as good. Instead of popping up when the character was speaking, these captions were late, often continuing after a scene had ended. Though flawed, it was still better than nothing.

After enjoying the full nine hours of the trilogy, we went to our local theater to see *The Hobbit*. The theater offers closed captioning at most shows. We chose a matinee and requested a closed caption device.

The device is a little screen on a long stalk that fits into the seat's cup holder. Three rows of text appear between shades that keep the light from bothering other patrons. The long bendy pole is meant to be super adjustable, but Julia is shorter than an adult (we've been teasing that she might actually BE a Hobbit). It was nearly impossible to get the thing to the right spot in her field of vision without blocking the movie screen. We spent a good ten minutes wrestling with the set up.

None of the previews were captioned. I kept checking expectantly, but the little display just said, "Captions are not available for this preview. Captioning will start with the feature presentation." Bummer.

Finally, the movie started. Julia was captivated. I could see her look to the captions frequently during scenes that were heavy on dialog. Afterwards, she said it was okay. Her main complaint was those shades that make the screen look dark unless it's angled just right. For some of the movie she actually held onto the screen to keep it tilted so she could see.

Though imperfect, captions have made life better. On our TV, we showed Julia how to turn them on herself. Now, most times we find her watching *Doc McStuffins* with the captions. She likes it and we've even convinced her that she can turn the volume down a bit.

Good news all around!

Walt Disney World Reflective Captioning
A Magic Ear Kids blog post from January 6, 2014:

Thanksgiving 2013 found our family crossing something off of my personal bucket list: Disney at Christmas. Ever since seeing an HGTV special on decorating the Magic Kingdom, I've wanted to go there. It was amazing! The castle covered in white lights was everything I dreamed it would be.

But there's only so long you can bask in the glow of Cinderella's castle. We spent time visiting other Orlando attractions as well as Hollywood Studios. It was there that we saw *Fantasmic* (billed as a "nighttime extravaganza") for the first time.

Using a combination of park maps and apps, we found that *Fantasmic* offers reflective captioning during the performance. We inquired at the entrance and were personally escorted by a staff member that set us up with the device.

Reflective captioning uses an acrylic glass panel to reflect the captions which are displayed (backwards of course) on a digital sign at the back of the amphitheater. We were seated in the "Mickey Mouse" section which was directly in front of the captioning display. Unfortunately, the staff member told us that we had to sit at the far end of the row. This placed a large pole between us and the caption display. Understanding, as we do, that a reflection requires a clear view of the thing you mean to reflect (you can't see your face in a mirror if your hand is in the way), we were skeptical. We had to wait to get it set up though because leading up to the show the screen was completely blank.

Once the show started, we scrambled to align the glass with the screen. We had to shift down the row to get that pole out of the way. It was a bit difficult as a parent because the reflection was only visible for our daughter. Sitting next to her it looked completely blank. It was a touch stressful!

After proper alignment was achieved, it worked wonderfully. Julia was able to understand parts of the show that were even a bit too garbled for her typically hearing parents. I heard Tim ask, "what did she say?" once during the show. Julia knew.

The next day in the Magic Kingdom, we again used reflective captioning for Mickey's *PhilharMagic.* We were again seated on the end of a row which put us in rather terrible seats for the 3D show. Once again, the screen was blank up until the show started. We hurried to set it up once the show began.

All in all, the reflective captioning was a great benefit for these shows. I'm not sure any of us are meant to understand Donald Duck, but according to the captions he is saying real words. My main suggestion to Disney would be to have a clear line of sight between the guest's seat and the caption screen. Also, it would be great if the screen could display something, even just an asterisk, to be lined up before the show starts. It's Disney magic - we don't want to miss a second!

SURFING AND OTHER POSSIBLE IMPOSSIBILITIES

Barbie in a Mermaid Tail is to blame for my daughter's surfing obsession. She watched that movie and immediately climbed atop this hand-me-down plastic seesaw in our yard, assumed a surfer's stance, and never stopped talking about it.

"Could I surf if Pittsburgh was closer to the ocean?" she'd ask.

"Um, sure. If Pittsburgh suddenly becomes coastal, I will take you surfing for sure."

The conversations were frequent and strangely demanding for a little girl so far inland. One day I told her, "surfing is really hard. You might not even be able to do it."

Usually a very supportive parent, I was really tired of what seemed like an impossible dream. As has been the case several times now in my parenting journey, within 18 months, Julia was making me eat my words.

August of 2012 found us off the northern coast of Oahu. We'd traveled with my husband on a work trip and found the North Shore Surf Girls to provide a lesson during our last day on the island.

Motherly commentary about her potential inability to "hang ten" ringing in her ears, Julia stood up on every wave. The surf instructor pulled her close to use basic signs and spoke loud enough to be heard while Julia was unaided.

After a couple hours on the water, they came ashore. Julia beamed with her accomplishment.

"She told me you said she wasn't going to be able to do that," the surf instructor said. "I think she showed you."

She really did.

Aside from the great surfing debacle of 2012, I've always been a mite over supportive my daughter conquering obstacles. I can remember one conversation where I excitedly explained the technology that doctors with hearing loss use to listen to a patient's heart through a stethoscope.

"Isn't that amazing? You could be a doctor!" I told her.
"But I don't want to be a doctor."
"Well, maybe not, but you could if you wanted to."

She sort of huffed and gave the grade school approximation of an eye roll.

Julia surfed many times after that. A year or so after our trip to Hawaii, I learned of Indo Jax Surf Charities from a Facebook post. The Wilmington, NC based surf school provides a series of surf camps for kids with hearing loss, visual impairments, autism, and other challenges. Given Julia's interest in surfing, I began stalking their website for information on the summer camps which are offered free of charge.

I began planning a trip to Wrightsville Beach seven months in advance. I need not have been so diligent (I might have placed a few phone calls) about securing Julia's spot in the camp. The owner, Jack, told the crowd of parents gathered that first year how it's very important that the surf school never has to turn kids away. Later that summer, 60 kids took part in the autism camp. I had been so worried that all the spots were going to be filled!

During the last week of July 2014, Julia and fourteen other kids with varying levels of hearing loss gathered at Mallard Street beach access #10 for several two-hour long sessions in the water. Instructors outnumbered participants and it soon became apparent that there was no need to worry about sending our little girl into the ocean. These guys, already having spent about eight hours in the ocean, were as attentive as Tim and I are with our own kid. As soon as Julia was off the board her instructor, Matt, was diving toward her. There was never a moment when any child was left to struggle even for a second. Parents walked back and forth on the shore, following their kids as the waves carried them down the beach.

She participated in the Indo Jax surf camp again the following summer. Surfers have long believed that theirs is not just a sport, but a transformative life event. Conquering the ever changing ocean instills a confidence unmatched by other pursuits. We could see it watching Julia during those evening surf sessions, her pride in standing up time after time.

Back on dry land, Julia really began to flourish in fifth and sixth grade. Her list of academic accomplishments is long. She's living a life without limits and that can be seen now equally on land and at sea. Though she hasn't been on a surfboard in a few years, I have to think that experience has done nothing but enforce her optimistic, can-do attitude. And she always has the memory of that time Mom really got it wrong.

CHASING THE WATERPROOF HEARING AID DREAM

Hearing aids and moisture don't mix. One of the first things our audiologist told us about Julia's little tan Phonak hearing aids was to keep them dry.

"Some of my sweaty boys ruin them just playing soccer," she told us.

We protected those things from every rain drop. School forms were emblazoned with the warning "WEARS HEARING AIDS THAT CANNOT GET WET." Julia eventually became so rain sensitive that you'd think she was going to melt. Every night the aids went into the high powered drying jar.

Water was a big concern and swimming was unaided.

After a few years, Julia upgraded to Phonak Naida aids. She chose light pink and we were relieved to learn they weren't quite as sensitive to moisture. Naida hearing aids were first advertised in a print ad where a mermaid wore a pair presumably thousands of leagues under the sea. By the time Julia's pair was dispensed they were classified as "water resistant." Quite a difference from mermaid-proof, but the added protection gave Julia the freedom of wearing them when her hair wasn't completely dry. Any spray park, pool, or water balloon fight action still had to be done unaided and communication was always a major issue.

Tim postulated that there ought to be some kind of waterproof receiver we could get to use in the pool. Even if it was a closed system with a microphone we'd wear. Our endless Internet searches never turned up anything more than waterproof headphones. Around 2013, we started seeing cochlear implant kids swimming with their devices.

We were jealous. Then we started seeing new ads for waterproof hearing aids.

Our audiologist advised that the claims of these new aids were perhaps a little exaggerated. (Maybe another mermaid ad situation.) Phonak Nios H20 hearing aids required a lot of maintenance after every exposure to water and swimming in every day hearing aids seems like too much risk. If the water hearing aids are also the school hearing aids, any water damage would derail school efforts. We needed to buy a second pair and had some difficulty figuring out how to do that for a pediatric patient.

So, we waited.

In the spring of 2014, a new round of research ensued as we anticipated swimming season. My husband found Siemens Aquaris aids with their IP 68 rating which he fully understands because he's an engineer.

This time around we even found a pediatric audiologist that would fit Julia for the aids. So, we embarked on a six-week trial with waterproof hearing aids.

We don't have them anymore.

From the beginning, the aids were plagued by frequent shut downs. We took them off of Julia and dried them, opened the battery door, and messed with them to get them to power on again. Sometimes they would be down for 15-20 minutes. On a swim trip with her Girl Scout troop, Julia took it upon herself to open the battery doors. In the water. She eventually decided she was happier without the hearing aids and swam for most of that day without them.

The audiologist (not our regular audiologist) indicated this was not normal performance for the instrument. We sent the aids back to Siemens for repairs. They replaced all of the guts and reported that there was evidence of water getting inside from opening the battery doors in the presence of water. Surprise! We started a new six-week trial and were instructed to pat the vent on the bottom of the batter door to dry it. This would allow the battery to breath and allow the hearing aid to turn on again. There was to be no opening of battery doors with wet hands or in the pool.

The experience with all the shutting down led to extensive research about hearing aid batteries by my husband, the resident scientist. He learned that the size 13 batteries we've been using for all these years are zinc air. This means the batteries need air to perform a reaction that creates the power needed to run hearing aids. We noticed for the first time ever that size 13 batteries have a little pin prick hole on the top. The sticker that comes on new batteries is keeping this hole closed, preserving the battery's power until it's ready for use. Some manufacturers recommend removing that sticker for a few minutes before putting the batteries in hearing aids. We've never had a problem with that, but a waterproof hearing aid isn't letting the battery breath when it's under water. Tim developed the hypothesis that these aids wouldn't shut down if we could use something other than a zinc air battery. He found rechargeable batteries that are nickel metal hydride and don't need air to work. We had hopes this would be our fix.

So, we tried again, very carefully, to swim with these hearing aids. The audiologist told us that Siemens does not endorse, recommend, or support the use of any rechargeable batteries in these hearing aids. Tim put the rechargeables in and the hearing aids turned on and worked for a whole day on dry land.

Problem solved?

No. That first time was some kind of fluke because on subsequent attempts, the hearing aids wouldn't power on with the rechargeable batteries. At least not every time. It was intermittent.

So that was a bummer, but we got one day at the pool with zinc air batteries that was pure bliss. Everything worked perfectly. Julia could hear, it was relaxing and blissful and everything we dreamed it would be. The aids shut off about four times, but we patted the special spot dry with a towel and continued about our day.

And that was it. Our one great shining moment. Julia got to swim three more times with the waterproof hearing aids. Shutting down became the least of our worries as constant debilitating feedback and distorted sound became the chief complaints. We found ourselves spending more time messing with the hearing aids than having fun in the pool. Julia decided that she was better off with no hearing aids at all while swimming.

Now we wait again for a hearing aid that is not only waterproof but entirely swimmable. The Siemens Aquaris aids most certainly are waterproof. You can dunk them in water and they still work flawlessly. Julia just spends too much time under water (they advertise these to be used for 30 minutes of submersion up to three feet deep) and perhaps she would do better if there was a pair of waterproof aids available in what they call "super power." At Julia's level of hearing loss, these aids were at full gain in the high frequencies. That means they were turned up as loud as they could go. Perhaps that had something to do with the performance issues.

Siemens discontinued the Aquaris hearing aid after just a few years. When Julia got her third pair of hearing aids, Phonak Sky in Caribbean blue, we downgraded the Naida aids to "swimming aids." She uses them for situations that might include a splash or a dunk. On one stand up paddle boarding trip, she fell into a lake with the pink Naidas. They survived the quick dunk and though they "don't sound as good" as her blue hearing aids, they're good enough for a canoe trip or a brief float on a pool noodle.

The waterproof hearing aids were a disappointment, but we learned a lot. I feel confident things are moving in the right direction. If not, maybe Julia won't always be so fond of being under the water. She might someday conquer a swimming pool the way I do: jump in and then shoulders up for the rest of the day. Water resistant devices are fine for that kind of pool trip.

THE LIFETONE SAFETY BEDSIDE FIRE ALARM

A Magic Ear Kids blog post from May 15, 2014:

Getting a smoke alarm for Julia has been on my list of things to do for quite some time. We don't currently leave her alone in the house, but it occurred to me that before long she'll be a teenager sleeping until noon and I might want to start my day before that. It will be necessary for her to independently wake up in case of emergency.

Much to my surprise, we were invited to sign up for a free Lifetone bedside fire alarm at a picnic for the Children's Hospital of Pittsburgh Hearing Center. A local Boy Scout, working toward his Eagle Scout Award, raised money to provide about sixty alarms for deaf and hard of hearing children in the area.

Just before Christmas, we received the bedside unit.

Not just a smoke alarm, this thing tells the date and time and acts as an alarm clock with a bed shaker, a little disk that rattles the bed so violently Julia could be thrown out!

This alarm does not detect smoke or fire on its own. It monitors the home for the other alarms. When it detects that specific sound, it triggers a 90dB sound as well as the bed shaker and a giant flashing display with the word "FIRE" in all caps. The household smoke detectors have to be T3 which means they give three tones then take a break. The Lifetone unit recognizes that pattern.

We unpackaged the new unit and followed the quick start guide. You simply plug it in and hit the test button on the nearest smoke alarm in the house. Our house alarms screeched. The Lifetone did nothing.

Turns out our existing smoke alarms were not T3. Our house is about seventeen years old. Smoke alarms, I learned from Google, should be replaced every ten years. We were overdue, and I wanted the kind that are both hard wired and battery. For some reason, I think my house is more likely to go up in flames when the electricity is out. This is probably irrational, but I still like a battery in my smoke alarm.

After replacing all our old alarms, the Lifetone worked flawlessly. It gives an added thrill when my kitchen activities inadvertently set off the smoke alarm on the first floor. The new alarms communicate with each other which in turn sets off that 90dB alarm and bed shaker. It's a big to-do when mom burns a pizza crust.

Julia wanted to try the alarm clock, so we set it one night. I went into her room a few minutes before it went off that morning to see what would happen.

When the alarm started, the bed shook so hard she rolled out and went stumbling away immediately. I laughed. It looked like she'd been ejected from the bed. We tried it on a subsequent morning and she was already immune. The 90dB horn blared, the bed shook, and she didn't even stir.

So, I think we need to schedule a middle of the night fire drill or consider training her to wake up for that sound. But having the Lifetone unit is a step toward peace of mind. I like that she'll be able to take it with her if she ever leaves home. Right now, we have it on good authority that she'll live with us forever. But, you know, it's a good option just in case.

CLASSMATES WITH HEARING LOSS, CO-TAUGHT CLASSROOMS & KNOWING WHEN IT'S TIME TO CHANGE UP THE TEAM

Hearing loss is a "low incidence disability" so we never expected Julia to encounter another person her age with a similar experience. We sought out other kids for her to play with in preschool and even organized a "magic ear playgroup" so she could have regular interaction with peers. She formed friendships with her magic ear group that had nothing to do with hearing loss. The parents benefited from sharing experiences, but the kids seemed unfazed by disability and unaware that their hearing loss put them in a minority. As grade school marched on, we saw less and less of the preschool support system, but it was good to know other kids existed and were close by if ever we felt alone.

By late elementary school, Julia was joined in her hearing support sessions by two other students. Just before the start of middles school, a fourth began using hearing aids. This is in a relatively rural, smallish school district that is patently homogeneous in all ways. That

Julia's grade would have so many kids with hearing loss was uncanny.

Over the years, Julia had become accustomed to one-on-one sessions with her itinerant teacher of the deaf. She worked through a curriculum that taught her all about conductive and sensorineural hearing losses. She'd begun instruction on assistive technology and had discontinued speech reading goals in favor of ASL by the time she was joined by these other students.

The addition of the new kids rolled back the clock on her program. Not only did she have to share her teacher, the lessons started back at the beginning. Julia was "teaching" about the causes of hearing loss. She wasn't spending much time at all learning ASL.

The relationship with the itinerant teacher was already on thin ice when the big move to sixth grade occurred. Steps were taken to smooth the transition to middle school in the same way we'd done with every grade, but as the years ticked by, starting a new school year morphed into a different sort of thing. At the beginning of every school year from kindergarten on, Julia and I would make a pilgrimage to her new classroom on the day before school started. These trips met with varying levels of success. Some teachers were welcoming and seemed glad to spend a few moments of their last day without students to talk through the FM system. They wanted to understand Julia's needs and have the most important parts of her IEP brought to their attention.

Other teachers preferred to figure things out as they

went along.

By fifth grade, it was obvious that teachers didn't want to talk to Mom anymore. About anything. Being gradually acclimated to my changing role as a parent, I accepted this as a natural part of having an older child.

At the start of the sixth-grade year, Julia went on her own to teach the building staff about her equipment.

It was an unmitigated disaster.

I'd had a call on the first day of summer vacation. The itinerant teacher of the deaf left a voicemail as we spent a family day at Idlewild, a nearby amusement park.

"Where are the FM receivers?" she wanted to know. "I'm checking in all of Julia's equipment and they're not here."

Now, we'd done things our own way throughout grade school. When she used the school-provided FM receivers, she would have to take them off and leave them at school overnight. This was causing her ears to become really red and irritated. The extra times in and out were just too rough on her skin. So rather than having Julia remove the school provided FM receivers every afternoon, we sent her to school with a pair that had been purchased through her own insurance. She wore them back and forth to school and didn't have to deal with rubbing her ears raw from taking her aids in and out each day.

This worked flawlessly for years. The receivers

purchased by the school remained safely at school in a case inside a shoebox of supplies and the receivers we owned went back and forth from home to school.

It bears mentioning that professionals and more experienced parents advised on multiple occasions that this was a bad idea.

At some point over the years, it may have been prior to fifth grade for all I know, the home receivers and the school receivers were swapped. Allegedly. These are identical Phonak receivers, but they have serial numbers printed on them in minuscule type. After fifth grade, the itinerant teacher checked and couldn't find the school receivers. Of course, the only explanation is that after so many years, we stole them.

I returned her call that summer day. I took a break from the merriment of Idlewild to let her know that we had our pair or receivers and there should be a pair in the box at school like always. I didn't hear any more about it until sixth grade in-service day.

As I positioned myself to await Julia's return from her talk with the new teachers, the itinerant teacher flew into the lobby. She was engaged in deep conversation with someone else, saw me, and practically screeched,

"DID YOU BRING THOSE RECEIVERS?"

"They should be in the box," I said. "We checked at home and we have one pair like always. I called you back this summer."

"I need to check the serial numbers," she said.

She proceeded to chastise me in front of other parents and the office staff for my family's carelessness with the school equipment.

"Those receivers cost a thousand dollars a pair," she said. "They'd better turn up."

At this point, I was unsure whether the receivers were lost, or it was just that they didn't have the correct serial number. I had ample time to think through all the options as I sat and stewed during the teacher meetings. My anger grew as I rehashed the conversation and the threat the teacher had leveled.

By the time the itinerant teacher breezed back to the school lobby with Julia and another student trailing behind, I felt hot under the collar. They returned without the shoebox in question and Julia had to be dispatched to retrieve it. Lo and behold, there were receivers in the box. The serial number issue turned out to be a non-issue. The great scandal was resolved, but the relationship with the itinerant teacher had gone from a teeter to the creaks and groans heard just before total collapse.

On the way home, Julia reported that she never wanted to meet her teachers in advance ever again.

"Mrs.--- called them all into one room. Then she told us to explain the FM to all of them at the same time. [The other students with hearing aids] wouldn't say a word. I had to explain everything. To all of them. At the same time. Mrs.--just stood there and sort of laughed at us."

School got underway and the complexity of the FM system with three students on it in various different classrooms overtaxed the ability of the professionals meant to coordinate it. At the same time, one of Julia's FM boots seemed to have died. We went through a long process to diagnose the problem and then order a new boot from her audiologist.

Julia came home in the first days of sixth grade with a copy of her schedule that was notated with various channels. To avoid interference, she was having to switch the FM transmitter channel almost every class. So, here's a brand-new sixth grader changing classes, memorizing a schedule and a locker combination, and dialing in a different FM channel for every class. The other students weren't changing channels. Presumably this was because Julia was the most experienced one in the group. This seemed invariably to bring all annoyance to her feet in an attempt to spare the others.

Tweaks were needed in those first days. One classmate would ask for the FM to be turned off during computer class. Turning the system off meant Julia didn't have it while the teacher read off letters of the alphabet for typing practice. The itinerant teacher intervened to inform everyone that they couldn't turn each other's FM off. Julia had her aids programmed with a mode to mute the FM, so she could quiet teachers as they helped other students.

We discovered soon after from Julia's reports that she

had a new Roger transmitter at school. A replacement for the FM transmitter she'd had since kindergarten, this would allow her finally to get boots with integrated receivers. The integrated receiver makes the overall length of the hearing aid less and adds increased water resistance to the whole device. The separate boot/receiver she typically used during the school year had diminished water resistance and did cause problems with moisture.

Tim is a technology guy. He was on eBay instantly and within a week had three different color options of Roger boots integrated with receivers as well as three different kinds of microphones that could transmit to the new receivers for use at home. He got a lapel mic, a Roger pen, and the same Roger transmitter being used at school.

As per usual, the involved parent is rewarded with disgust and bureaucracy. The itinerant teacher and the audiologist the school contracted with couldn't figure out how to integrate this change into the already dysfunctional system they'd developed. One particular issue was deemed unresolvable. Julia's World Geography class was co-taught and there was no way to mic both teachers. Having only one transmit to Julia's hearing aids made it very difficult to hear the other. Additionally, Julia's Roger transmitter could send a signal to the other student's hearing aid using a regular FM receiver, but the FM transmitter the other student used could not transmit a signal to Julia's integrated Roger receivers.

The world was surely ending there for a while.

After a couple of weeks in contact with various different professionals multiple times per day, I was sure that the best thing would be for my husband to go and set everything up using the knowledge he'd obtained from the Phonak web site. For some reason, it seemed he was the only one that could read the Roger instruction manual. Conversations with the school audiologist revealed severe gaps in her understanding of the equipment. It was near torture.

Upon reaching wit's end, I began emailing with the classroom teacher in that co-taught World Geography class. A co-taught classroom is where the students have two licensed teachers rather than one. It's akin to the classrooms that have a special education paraprofessional, but the co-teacher has other classes where she's the only educator. It's a method of providing extra support for students with special needs.

"I looked at Julia's schedule," the teacher wrote. "I have a class with only twelve students first period. Julia has study hall then. Why don't we just switch her to that class? It doesn't have a co-teacher."

The hallelujah chorus played when I opened that email! The scheduling change was made, and we entered a long period of enjoying the consistent workhorse that is the Roger system. Sixth grade began to gain momentum.

The horror of the first weeks behind us, reports began coming home of the itinerant teacher's fixation on the safety of the equipment.

"Better not lose that," she'd call out passing in the hallway.

Pull out sessions became the most stressful part of Julia's day. The teacher would miss seeing Julia in study hall and make her late for her next class. We came to realize that the stresses of middle school weren't being caused by middle school. The itinerant hearing support was causing more harm than good.

It was an uncomfortable phone call to make. The itinerant teacher seemed to grasp the gravity of the situation. We were essentially firing her. I made the request that her services be reduced from two short pull-out sessions per week and one push-in to consultation only. This meant she wouldn't interact with Julia anymore.

Removing the itinerant support was an important decision and it had an immediate effect. Julia was more at ease in school. We realized her interactions with that teacher had been difficult for a long time. Instead of support, it had become obligation.

Having a long, established history makes it all the more difficult to make a change in the support team. Sometimes it's necessary though. In this case, the best way forward was to reduce level of school provided support and to let Julia have more of the independence she's worked so hard to earn.

The tumultuous beginning of sixth grade calmed to a

predictable routine and as middle school marches on I don't hear much about the other kids with hearing loss. The Roger system works all of the time. By now the school should be more adept at these accommodations.

ON SOMETIMES AVOIDING MESSES

The hearing aids can't get wet. This might be the first thing we taught Julia about her "magic ears" and over the course of the first two years, I succeeded in making her perfectly terrified of rain, children with squirt guns, and even the grocery store produce shelf misting nozzles. In retrospect, maybe I overdid it. Still, she learned early that the hearing aids are important, and she diligently took care of them starting at an early age.

Other hazards introduced themselves and warnings were issued about sunscreen, hair spray, and face creams. By fourth grade we realized that life would occasionally throw weird destructive opportunities into the mix.

At least once a year in K-4, I volunteered for one of the seasonal parties. A sign-up sheet at open house set a schedule for the year. In kindergarten, I invited all the moms to my house for a planning session. The primary school parent scene gently let me figure out that planning wasn't meant to be that involved. By the fourth grade Winter Break party, I just showed up with a craft of my own choosing.

Craft time was followed by a series of game stations. I was positioned out in the hall within smelling distance of a clogged toilet. (These stories are making my daughter's school sound awful, overall, it's not that bad.)

Since I was put in charge of the cup stacking game, I really just had to reign in the rambunctious boys that were past ready for school to end for winter break. I turned my attention to a friend from church that was setting up another station.

She spread a vinyl table cloth on the floor and began unloading shower caps and shaving cream.

"What are they going to do here?" I asked.
"Oh, it's so fun," she said. "You put shaving cream on the shower cap and then you throw cheese curls at the shaving cream to try to get them to stick."
"And the point of this is?"
"Well, they're white cheese. So, at the end you're supposed to look like Frosty the Snowman."

Julia appeared at my station in the first group of kids. She still liked having me around in those days.

"You're going to have to give Mrs. R's thing a wide berth I think. If someone gets shaving cream on your hearing aids I will have to kill them. And it's almost Christmas."

She stacked cups and then stood with me until her group finished coating themselves with shaving cream. We watched together and decided it didn't look like that much fun.

The hearing aids come first in all things. They were carefully tucked under a bandana during the chalk dusting of a Color Vibe 5K. They've been safely in a dry bag for all water activities. She's skipped two rounds of something called "Messy Olympics" at youth group and never lets anyone pass a soaking sponge over her head. It's brought a different level of awareness to our lives. She won't be volunteering to take a banana crème pie to the face. The hearing aids are an excuse to occasionally avoid messes.

EAR MOLD MANIA

Once upon a time, the most taxing part of getting new ear molds was the color selection. Julia would pour over the samples and a laminated card of color choices while the bright green-yellow impression material hardened in each ear. She insisted on having the impressions taken one ear at a time, so she didn't miss anything that was being said. Decision time came, and she still wouldn't be ready to commit. Choosing up to four colors that could be striped, swirled, polka dotted, or floated in an abyss of clear silicone, the possibilities were endless.

When she was about eight, we started having trouble with the fit of the ear molds. The molds were mailed to us to expedite the process. They arrived and looked visibly different from the usual shape. We wondered if these were even from Julia's impressions.

The ear mold manufacturer keeps impressions around for a week or so. We called the audiologist and were sent a new pair. They still weren't right. And so, we embarked on a maddening process of new impressions and phone calls and even in-person visits to the ear mold making facility. We tried the other audiologist that fitted the swimming hearing aids. We had open mouth impressions. Tim took detailed measurements and produced drawings that only an engineer could make.

Eventually, Children's Hospital of Pittsburgh authorized our audiologist to send impressions to the facility that makes ear molds for UPMC's adult patients. Months passed, and we were notified that those impressions got lost in the mail.

There are two ear mold manufacturing facilities in the country. We tried both. Both failed.

To bridge the gap while waiting for the rest of the world to get their ear mold act together, we took to sifting through old ear molds to find some that would fit. Julia settled on the royal blue and purple set that came with her swimming hearing aids. She wore those until they hardened into rock-like lumps that could no longer suppress the feedback.

Out of the blue, a pair of ear molds arrived from Colorado. The lost impressions were found! The ear molds weren't perfect, but they didn't squeal. The ear mold mania subsided for another year.

Though Julia's ears aren't growing anymore, ear molds only last a year. The constant drying of the hearing aid dehumidifier causes them to harden. Eventually they lose some mass. They cease to be comfortable. They squeal.

It took two attempts with the most recent impressions

to get passable molds. These are a far cry from what we were getting in the first five years of hearing aid use. The prevailing professional theory is that Julia is more discerning about the feel of the ear molds now that she's older.

I'm not so sure. Her hearing aids are a high enough power that the fit needs to be very tight. Around the time we started having trouble, we found out the facility switched from making the molds by hand to using an automated process. The quality seems to have degraded significantly. If feedback weren't such an issue, a hearing aid user might not notice. Unfortunately, Julia notices.

And so, we keep fighting and remolding. Eventually, the earmold factory might re-learn how to do that which we took for granted in the beginning. If they don't, we're going to accumulate a whole lot of odd looking ear molds.

TURNS OUT THE PINK HEARING AIDS CAN TAKE SOME ABUSE

Technology trickles down in our family. The newest and best thing comes into the house and pushes the old version down the line. It might be sold or given to the kid or used as a backup. This has happened with CD players and iPods and iPhones. Even hearing aids have entered the family electronics funnel.

When Julia got her pink Naida hearing aids, the little tan eXtra 311 aids became her back up pair. We tried having her wear them on a trip to Lake Erie. Encased in hot pink Ear Gear (a protective covering purchased online) they were protected from sand, but the sound was muffled. The Ear Gear caused excessive feedback and the beach was more enjoyable without hearing aids. By that time, her hearing loss had moved into the severe range and the old ones weren't loud enough even without the Ear Gear.

It was really the third pair of hearing aids, the bright blue Phonak Sky pair, that made it possible to have a true backup. Julia notices a significant difference in the sound quality, but after the Siemens waterproof aids failed, she took to wearing the Naidas in potential water hazard situations. Affectionately called "the pinkies," she's worn them on water slides, in lazy rivers, and most frequently, stand up paddle boarding. Unlike surfing, stand up paddle boarding (SUP) the calm water of the streams and lakes near Pittsburgh doesn't pose much risk of submersion. The idea is to stand up on the board. With Julia wearing the pink hearing aids, we can cruise around and talk about the sights. She can get far from us and still hear if we warn her she's about to run into a boat.

Our first SUP experience was a lesson and eco-tour on Lake Arthur at Moraine State Park. The instructor led our group in a round of SUP dodgeball after we were comfortable on the boards. This involved using the paddle to fling a sponge at each other. If the sponge landed on your board, you were out. Our group wasn't very aggressive, but in the melee, Julia fell in. She bobbed to the surface quickly thanks to her life vest. I held my breath and we paddled over to her. Would the pinkies survive?

A few tense moments ensued, but after a bit of dabbing with what dry material we could find, the pinkies returned to normal. They survived momentary full submersion. Perhaps the mermaid ad wasn't so far off after all.

The aids took a second dip in the intracoastal waterway of North Carolina during another SUP excursion. They worked consistently the entire time, unaffected by the water.

According to the IP rating, the Phonak Sky aids should be even more water resistant than the Naidas. We've never been comfortable putting her main hearing aids at risk that way. Hopefully, the pinkies will keep working for our water adjacent activities. It does improve our family life to have such easy communication on the water.

THINGS THAT GO BUZZ IN THE NIGHT

The Lifetone bedside fire alarm brought us some peace of mind although we've still never left Julia alone while she's sleeping. She's never learned to wake herself with the alarm clock portion of the device, so I remain skeptical that it would rouse her in a fire.

She once set the alarm accidentally. Awakened by the 90-dB alarm honking, the buzzing bed shaker, and a general sense of horrified anxiety, I raced into her room. She was sleeping peacefully, completely undisturbed by the flashing and whirring of the little unit. At some point in the six years before college, we're going to need to figure out something that works.

In the meantime, we've had the Lifetone unit there at the ready.

The alarm just sort of hung out on her bedside table, listening and quietly doing its job until one afternoon this obnoxious racket issued forth from Julia's bedroom. It was buzzing and vibrating in a pattern. When I got to the room, the screen was flashing,

"BED!" Lifting the mattress off the bed shaker disc quieted the machine. The display returned to normal.

This happened occasionally every few months. I determined it was because shaker disc was being used on a daybed. This caused it to be positioned between a mattress and a hard board and obviously made it unhappy. It would freak out and I would go shift things around to pacify it again. It never occurred to me that this malfunction could and would eventually take place in the dead of night.

It was 12:38am when the buzzing started. My husband snores and I'd fled the marital bed chamber years before to sleep in the blissful quiet of our spare room. Since this shares a wall with Julia's room, the vibrations sounded like the apocalypse. I shot into her room in the dark and began clawing at the alarm.

I'd been asleep since 10:15pm. I'm not sure I gained full consciousness until several moments into my frenzied dig to suppress this awful noise. The alarm possesses the capacity to set off every smoke alarm in the house. The thing was practically a bomb. Pull the wrong wire and the whole house was going to erupt in a cacophony of beeps. It wasn't possible to lift the mattress and free the bed shaker with Julia in the bed. I couldn't figure out how to make it stop.

I left the buzzing and opened my husband's door.

"I'm having trouble with Julia's alarm clock, can you help me?"

He was up and out of bed immediately. We worked together to silence the shaking. Morning found the alarm with every cord unplugged in a pile with four "D" cell batteries. We weren't taking any chances of it returning to life.

In the morning, I consulted the owner's manual. This might have been a worthwhile step all those months before. I determined the bed shaker wasn't going to work and reinstalled the unit without it.

Now I look forward to being awakened by just the 90-dB honking in the night. It's got to be better than the buzz!

ADULTS SAY THE DARNDEST THINGS

You wouldn't know…

People have a hard time knowing what to say. I get this because I am a person. I don't always say the right thing and I surely don't always even know what the right thing might have been. Still, I'd be remiss to leave out our experience of the public perception of moderate-to-severe hearing loss, hearing aids, and to a lesser extent, disability. The silly things people say are part of the experience.

The most frequent comment I hear is some form of "you wouldn't even know there's anything, you know…. with her."

Notably and blessedly absent from this comment is the word "wrong" because that's what the speaker is searching for in those stumbling mid-sentence moments.

"You wouldn't even know there's anything wrong with her."

This comes up when the hearing aids are brought to the attention of someone that already knew about them, but hasn't been called on to think of the daily implications or accommodations needed. It's a response to a mention of the hearing aids not being able to get wet or how sounds don't bother her at night or that it's tough to have a conversation in the pool.

To analyze this statement is to become pretty annoyed. Angry even. There isn't anything "wrong" with her. Except maybe the usual things, the things that are "wrong" with us all.

I try to avoid feeling at odds with our friends and family, so I've reframed this as a compliment. I choose to hear the meaning underneath as, "Gosh, I'm surprised. She does so well and having hearing loss really doesn't limit her in any way."

This way it makes sense when I respond, "thanks, she does very well."

Can she hear me?

Less common, but not entirely infrequent is the person that sees the hearing aids and begins making all sorts of assumptions. It's as if they get out their jump to conclusions mat and begin a wild hop through all of the possibilities.

In the summer after sixth grade, Julia was invited to present her award winning history project at the site of the battle that was the subject of her project. She stood in a crowded room and gave a brief overview of her research. Afterward, she stood by her display and answered questions.

This was an extremely difficult listening environment. The building was old and had those open floor plan miserable acoustics that magnify even the quietest side conversation. People were milling around and there were a million different conversations going on at once. Tim and I were by Julia's side to help if there were issues with hearing the people that came to talk to her. All three of us struggled, as did the rest of the people in the room.

An older woman approached us, took a quick look at Julia then turned to me and said, "Can she hear me? Does she read lips?"

It wasn't the time or the place to point out how very rude it is to have a conversation about someone when they're standing right next to you. We indicated that Julia can in fact hear and her lip reading ability, though very limited, wasn't especially relevant at the moment.

ASL

Later in the summer, a distant cousin asked Julia in sign language if she signs.

"Your weird cousin was signing at me," she told me as we drove home from a brief appearance at a family event. "He asked me if I sign and said that he's self-taught."
"What did you say?"
"I said 'I sign a little' and 'good for you' and I walked away."

She spoke these words to the cousin. Our attempts at learning ASL have met with little success. We had a family discussion about this new variation of the hearing loss response. It was the first time a person outside of an educational or support group environment used or talked about ASL. It was a surprise.

Our opinions varied between "nice and thoughtful gesture" and "complete cultural ignorance." Of course, being the most negative thinker in the family, my take on it was the latter. Having spent so much time with other families of kids with hearing loss and learning about Deaf culture, I thought the cousin might have really stepped in it if the person he signed at was a staunch oral education proponent.

Perhaps the deeper issues lie in the awkwardness of large family events, but I think it's always best to engage in a normal bit of conversation. If it's impossible to keep your ASL knowledge to yourself, bring it up after you're through the stranger danger phase.

The Right Way

The good news is everyday there are people that handle hearing loss and those highly visible, wildly colored hearing aids the right way. They ignore them. They acknowledge, even if it's subconscious, that Julia probably doesn't want to talk about it all the time. She likely doesn't think about it every waking moment. She is normal. You can be normal too.

TAKING CREDIT WHETHER I DESERVE IT OR NOT

In Pennsylvania, the wonderful medical assistance pays for eight hearing aid batteries per calendar month. A pair of batteries lasts about one week, so the insurance covers an ample allotment. Of course, the round button batteries have found their way into every crevice of our home and cars. Countless bedding searches and sojourns under furniture with flashlight have turned up all but the most ornery. Having eight batteries per month provides a cushion for the days when they seem to do nothing but drop and roll.

The insurance provided batteries have been a great benefit over the years, but it's become harder to use now that we're not visiting Children's Hospital or its satellite offices on a regular basis. The monthly batteries can't be mailed. They must be picked up in person.

When Julia was having private speech therapy, I'd walk around the front of the Children's North building and collect the batteries once per month. This sometimes took longer than her speech therapy appointment because there was a sign in sheet that put battery pickups into the same queue as the patients seeing a host of other doctors. Then, once called to the window and stating a need for batteries, the receptionist had to go back into the audiologist's office to dig two packs of size 13s out of the closet.

It was such a drawn out process, I couldn't count on being done with it during Julia's speech therapy appointment. I'd have to take her with me to collect batteries before or after. Each time, I wondered why they couldn't just have the batteries at the counter. It was an inefficient process and obviously as irritating to the staff as it was for me.

Sometime later, a postcard mailer showed up (or maybe an email) requesting feedback on Children's Hospital of Pittsburgh. I was a marketing major in college and I'll take a market research survey about anything. I complain and praise and review. I was glad to tell Children's what I think.

Though there wasn't a truly appropriate place on the questionnaire, I was sure to insert my experience with picking up batteries. I suggested that the battery supply could be moved to the front desk area.

The very next month, we signed in and were thrilled to have batteries produced from easy reach of the receptionist. The lengthy process was already more efficient.

"I did that," I thought.

The pickup procedure has evolved significantly since then. There's now a separate sign in binder for batteries and today we can walk into Children's North and head home with two packs of PowerOne hearing aid batteries in under five minutes.

There's really no way to know if it was my suggestion that forever changed the Children's Hospital battery dispensing protocol, but occasionally, I like to take a little credit whether I deserve it or not. Parenting doesn't offer much opportunity for accolades. I might have put my daughter in a position to successfully learn to speak, but I couldn't do the work for her. The achievement is hers alone. She talks and reads and comprehends. I was there, but I can't take the credit.

And so, I pat myself on the back for the battery thing. Yeah, I did that.

TROUBLESHOOTING AND MOM FIXES THAT AVOID A TRIP TO THE AUDIOLOGIST

The first pair of hearing aids were scary. The audiologist showed us how to put in the batteries and wiggle them into little ears. My husband is a technological genius and might have taken to programming the aids himself were it not such a critical part of my daughter's wellbeing. For me, the inner workings were a miraculous mystery. Even from different spheres of understanding, both parents were on the same page: if anything went wrong, we high-tailed it to the professional.

"I can have these molds sent right to your house and you can cut the tubes," we were told after one appointment for impressions. "You can probably do it just as well as I can."

The new ear molds arrived about ten days later. I carefully measured and cut with shaking hands, nervous because there's no going back if the tubes end up too short. They can be replaced, but it's never as good as those first tubes with the grommets firmly wedged inside. The first try ended up a little long, but by carefully shaving them down, little by little, tube perfection was achieved. My confidence with handling the aids increased.

Now, outfitted with a kit of commonly needed supplies, there's a full service of "mom fixes" that the hearing aids go through before making a special trip to the audiologist. The following is a troubleshooting guide based on our completely unprofessional experience with Phonak Naida and Sky hearing aids. If you're uncomfortable handling the hearing aids, consult with your pediatric audiologist.

Problem	Solution
Squealing/ Feedback	Three things can cause incessant feedback that doesn't stop when the hearing aid is firmly inserted, and nothing is interfering with it (as in hats, hair, or a cozy hug): 1. A hole in the tubing – the best way to test for this is to remove the hearing aid, cover the hole in the ear mold and wiggle the tube. If the hearing aid squeals, there's a hole in the tubing. Remove the old tube and insert a new one. 2. Gunk on the speaker covers – this is difficult to see, so I routinely replace the little grey spongey pads when there's any issue with sound quality or feedback. It's also important to avoid getting hair gel or sunscreen on these pads. The replacement covers have a small, pointy tool for poking out the old

	ones and pushing the new into place. I try to put the sticky side down to avoid picking up dust, but it's a tricky procedure and sometimes whichever direction it happens to end up in wins. 3. Ear molds are not fitting tight enough – over time, even when the child is done growing, ear molds dry out and harden. Squealing is the #1 sign that it's time to head to the audiologist for new impressions. Just be sure to check for a hole in the tube before you make the appointment!
Muffled/ Quiet Operation	1. Change the batteries – new batteries are a game changer with all kinds of odd reports. No matter what the concern, it never hurts to try a fresh pair of batteries. 2. Change those speaker covers – see #2 in the squealing/feedback section. Debris on those covers can mute the sound a bit. 3. Clean the ear mold tubing – wax builds up in the tubing on a regular basis. Occasionally, a drop of moisture will impact sound quality. We've found grains of sand in there. Remove the tubing from the hearing aid and clean the tube with water. Look for the bulby air blower in your supply kit to blow the moisture out of the tubes. 4. Change the ear hooks – Both the Sky and Naida hearing aids have a little mini tiny cotton ball in the ear

	hook part of the aid. It's some sort of filter and after years of use with both sets of hearing aids, it becomes a problem. In the Naida aids, this filter would become visibly blown up and the hearing aid would essentially be muted. In the Sky aids, the filter looks fine, but there was all kinds of crackling. We spent a full summer of audiology and ENT to figure out it was just the ear hook filter. Unscrew the old ear hook and tighten on a new one.
Unexplained Beeping	Before switching to Roger integrated receivers, both the Naidas and Sky hearing aids went through periods of unexplained beeping. The Sky aids are prone to playing a long, musical song when they're unhappy. We found this to be caused by the FM boots. Removing the boots resolved the beeping. Unfortunately, you may need a trip to the audiologist for new boots.
Any Complaint Whatsoever Not Listed Above	Full in-home hearing aid service: change batteries, replace ear mold tubing, new hooks, new speaker covers, and assurances, "I've done everything I can do." If that doesn't work, call in the pros!

PRODUCTS AND EQUIPMENT

The following is a list of products and equipment we've tried for Julia's hearing aids. Some things have worked well, others not so much.

Hal-Hen ® Super Dri-Aid ™: This is the first hearing aid dehumidifier we purchased. It does a fine job. This is currently the home of the pink Naida hearing aids and the drying jar used for travel. The desiccant balls need to be microwaved periodically to restore their moisture capturing capability. Some of the balls turn bright blue in color when they've been sufficiently refreshed.
http://www.halhen.com

Dry and Store Global II Electric Hearing Aid Dehumidifier: A few years ago, we upgraded to this plug-in drying box with a UV sanitizing lamp. We've had to replace the lightbulb once in spite of assurances from the manufacturer that the bulb lasts longer than the unit. Desiccant blocks must be replaced every two months. They're available on amazon.com in a six pack.
http://dryandstore.com/

Ear Gear: A spandex nylon sleeve that covers behind the ear hearing aids and cochlear implant processors to provide protection from sweat, dirt, and moisture. It's also supposed to cut down on wind noise. Julia's hearing aids are quite high

powered and using Ear Gear caused intolerable feedback. Ear Gear didn't work for her.
https://www.gearforears.com/

Power One Batteries: Julia uses Power One zinc air batteries. When she's using her Roger system at school, a pair of batteries lasts one week. Battery life is shown to be a bit longer if the sticker is removed for five minutes before putting the battery in the hearing aid. We also have a pair of "eco-friendly NiMH batteries" that were purchased during the Siemens Aquaris trial period. These worked well but are not recommended for use in any of Julia's current hearing aids.

Phonak: Julia has had three pairs of Phonak hearing aids. She's likely to stay with Phonak in the future as different companies have varying technologies for sound compression and amplification that cause differences in the hearing experience. She likes the way Phonak aids sound.

Roger: From phonakpro.com… "Roger is the digital standard, providing outstanding performance in noise and over distance by wirelessly transmitting a speaker's voice directly to the listener. It offers a staggering breakthrough in signal-to-noise ratio and guarantees access to new levels of speech understanding." Advertised as being better, clearer, and easier than traditional FM systems, Julia's been using Roger for a little over a year. It's working perfectly! Check eBay for affordable refurbished and demo equipment. We were able to get the Inspiro transmitter, Roger Pen, lapel mic, and several pairs of integrated receivers for under $400.

Telecoil Ear Hooks: Simple, reliable technology for listening to any audio source with a standard headphone jack. Julia has MusicLink brand ear hooks. Amazon is selling NoiZfree Audio Binaural Earhooks now which is the same technology, but we have no experience with that brand. Hearing aids do need to have a telecoil mode enabled to use these "headphones."

Lifetone HLAC Fire Alarm and Clock: easy to use and portable, the Lifetone bedside fire alarm listens for your household smoke detectors and blasts a loud alarm when it "hears" their signal. This alarm is still with us because it's all we have at present. It doesn't wake Julia and we've had to discontinue use of the bed shaker.
http://lifetonesafety.com/

Resources

Alexander Graham Bell Association for the Deaf and Hard of Hearing -- http://www.agbell.org/, 3417 Volta Place, NW | Washington, DC 20007, (202) 337-5220

American Society for Deaf Children – http://www.deafchildren.org/, 800 Florida Avenue, NE #2047, Washington, DC 20002-3695, (800)942-2732

Hands & Voices -- http://www.handsandvoices.org/, PO Box 3093, Boulder, CO 80307, (303) 492-6283

ABOUT THE AUTHOR

Joey Lynn Resciniti lives North of Pittsburgh, Pennsylvania with her husband, their only-child, Julia, and the family's two shih tzus. She maintains the blog, Magic Ear Kids (http://magicearkids.blogspot.com), as a resource for parents of children with hearing loss. She writes about other aspects of family life more regularly on the Big Teeth & Clouds blog (http://bigteethclouds.blogspot.com).

Joey published a work of fiction in the summer of 2017 titled, No Room for Hondo.

82937044R00104

Made in the USA
Columbia, SC
21 December 2017